The Zero Rupee Upanishad

RAJAT AKRE

ISBN: 978-93-344-5610-3

DEDICATION

To everyone who ever tried to buy peace on Amazon.

To everyone who thought enlightenment came with a 7-day free trial.
And to the ancient sages who gave away cosmic secrets for free,
you'd be cancelled today for "undermining the wellness industry."

This book costs nothing, except the paper you're holding.
The wisdom, as always, is free — straight from the Source.

CONTENTS

ACKNOWLEDGMENTS

I owe this book to every overpriced wellness ad that made me angry enough to write it.

To the sun, for showing up every morning without asking for a sponsorship.
To air, water, and gravity for not charging subscription fees (yet).
To my students, who kept asking for "the secret to life" , here it is, and it costs zero rupees.

You're only paying for the ink and paper that trapped these free ideas inside a rectangle.

The wisdom itself remains open-source, courtesy of the universe, which still runs the most generous free plan ever designed.

CHAPTER 1: SUNLIGHT

The Sun Never Sets on Our Vitamin D Deficiency (Welcome to Peak Irony)

Picture this: You're standing in the queue at your nearest chai tapri at 2 PM on a blazing Delhi afternoon, the sun beating down mercilessly as you sweat through your third shirt change of the day. The UV index is probably somewhere between "mildly carcinogenic" and "surface of Mercury," and you're mentally calculating how much of your monthly salary went toward that fancy Japanese sunscreen your dermatologist swore by. Meanwhile, your mom calls—again—to inform you that your latest blood test shows Vitamin D deficiency and you need to "get more sunlight."

Welcome to India in the 21st century, where we have abundant sunshine approximately 300 days a year, yet 70-90% of us are somehow Vitamin D deficient. It's like living next to a five-star buffet and still managing to be malnourished. But before you blame this entirely on our collective obsession with fair skin (thanks, matrimonial ads and Bollywood), or our newfound love affair with air-conditioned offices, let's talk about what sunlight actually *is*, what it does, and why our relationship with it has become more complicated than a Karan Johar movie plot.

The Physics of Solar Radiation (Or: How the Sun Became Your Friendly Neighborhood Nuclear Reactor)

Let's start with the basics, because understanding sunlight means understanding one of the universe's most elegant energy delivery systems. At its core—literally—the Sun is a massive nuclear fusion reactor sitting 150 million kilometers away, converting hydrogen into helium and releasing absurd amounts of energy in the process. Thanks to Einstein's famous $E=mc^2$, even tiny amounts of mass lost in this fusion translate into enormous energy output. Every second, the Sun converts about 4 million tons of matter into pure energy. Yes, tons. Every second.

This energy travels to Earth as electromagnetic radiation, which is just a fancy physics term for waves of electric and magnetic fields oscillating through space at the speed of light. Think of it like the ultimate wireless power transmission system—no cables, no monthly bills, just 93 million miles of vacuum and a consistent 1,366 watts per square meter hitting the top of Earth's atmosphere.

But here's where it gets interesting for those of us stuck in Delhi's smog or Mumbai's humidity: not all sunlight is created equal, and definitely not all of it reaches you while you're trying to get that perfect Instagram shot at Marine Drive.

The Electromagnetic Spectrum: A Rainbow on Steroids

Sunlight isn't just one type of light—it's a cocktail of different wavelengths of electromagnetic radiation. About 44% of the Sun's energy that reaches Earth falls within the visible light spectrum, the range our eyes can actually detect, roughly between 400 and 700 nanometers. This is your classic VIBGYOR (because we're Indian and we learned Roy G. Biv backward in school).

But visible light is just the opening act. The full solar spectrum includes:

Ultraviolet (UV) radiation (100-400 nm): The troublemaker of the family. UV radiation is subdivided into UVA (315-400 nm), UVB (280-315 nm), and UVC (100-280 nm). UVC gets filtered out completely by Earth's ozone layer—thank goodness, because it's nasty stuff. UVB is what gives you sunburns and triggers Vitamin D synthesis (yes, the same chemical process). UVA penetrates deeper into your skin, causes aging, and despite what your neighborhood aunty says about "harmless tanning," it's strongly linked to melanoma.

Visible light (400-700 nm): This is what allows you to see your reflection in the metro window and judge whether your hair survived the Bangalore traffic. Different wavelengths within this range produce different colors—violet and blue at the shorter end (400-500 nm), green in the middle, and red at the longer end (625-750 nm).

Infrared radiation (700 nm - 1 mm): The invisible heat you feel. This is why standing in sunlight feels warm even on a winter morning in Shimla. About 49% of solar radiation reaching Earth is infrared. Your skin absorbs this radiation, molecules start vibrating faster, and boom—you feel warm. It's the same principle behind those infrared heaters, except the Sun's version has been around for 4.6 billion years and doesn't increase your electricity bill.

Here's the physics equation that governs all of this: $E = hf = hc/\lambda$, where E is photon energy, h is Planck's constant (6.626×10^{-34} J·s), f is frequency, c is the speed of light, and λ is wavelength. This relationship tells us something crucial: shorter wavelengths pack more energy. That's why UV radiation can damage your DNA (high energy, short wavelength), while infrared just makes you feel toasty (lower energy, longer wavelength).

The Indian Solar Reality Check

Now, India is blessed—or cursed, depending on whom you ask and what month it is—with tremendous solar potential. The country lies in the tropical region with the Tropic of Cancer literally passing through it, giving us high solar insolation and approximately 300 sunny days per year. Our solar potential is estimated at 748 GW, and we've already installed over 127 GW of solar capacity as of 2025.

But here's the catch that nobody warned you about in your engineering thermodynamics class: India is also getting *dimmer*. Yes, you read that right. Despite having abundant sunshine, the actual amount of sunlight reaching the ground has been declining for the past 30 years.

A comprehensive study analyzing data from 20 weather stations between 1988 and 2018 found that sunshine hours have steadily decreased across most of India. In northern inland areas—your Amritsars and Kolkatas—annual sunshine reductions have been most significant. Mumbai's sunshine hours have been gradually declining too.

The culprit? Aerosols and air pollution.

Those tiny particles from vehicle emissions, industrial output, and agricultural burning act as nuclei for cloud formation, making clouds denser and longer-lived, effectively blocking more sunlight. Aerosols have reduced ground-level sunlight by about 13%, while clouds add another 31-44% reduction in surface solar radiation. It's like India wrapped itself in a pollution blanket and now wonders why it feels darker.

The irony is nuclear-level here: we're investing billions in solar infrastructure while simultaneously choking our own skies with pollution that reduces solar panel efficiency by 12-41%, costing an estimated $245-835 million in lost power generation. It's the renewable energy equivalent of buying a gym membership and then eating samosas in the parking lot.

The Biochemistry of Sunshine (Or: What Actually Happens When Light Hits Your Face)

The Vitamin D Saga: India's Paradoxical Deficiency

Let's address the elephant in the room—or rather, the sunshine in the sky that we're somehow not benefiting from. India has a Vitamin D deficiency crisis of epic proportions. Studies show that 70-90% of Indians are Vitamin D deficient despite living in a sun-drenched country. This is roughly equivalent to a fish being dehydrated.

The mechanism is beautifully simple: when UVB photons (wavelengths 280-315 nm) hit your skin, they interact with 7-dehydrocholesterol, a cholesterol derivative present in your skin cells. This photochemical reaction converts it into pre-vitamin D_3, which then undergoes a temperature-dependent isomerization to become vitamin D_3. Your liver and kidneys then convert it into the active form your body can use.

Research from Tirupati (latitude 13.40° N) using an in vitro model showed that the best conversion of 7-dehydrocholesterol to active vitamin D happens between 11 AM and 2 PM, when the solar zenith angle is optimal. During this window, conversion rates hit around 11.5%. Studies from Delhi demonstrated that serum vitamin D increases by 2.03 ng/mL per hour of sun exposure (95% CI: 1.77-2.28).

So why are we still deficient? The reasons form a perfect storm of modern lifestyle and traditional preferences:

1. Cultural attitudes toward skin color: Let's not dance around this. Fairness creams are a multi-billion rupee industry in India. The matrimonial section still lists "wheatish complexion" as a compromise between honesty and desirability. People actively avoid sunlight to maintain fair skin.

2. Urbanization and indoor lifestyles: Agricultural workers in rural India have vitamin D levels around 24 ng/mL, while urban dwellers average 19 ng/mL. We've traded outdoor work for air-conditioned offices. The IT professional in Bangalore sees less sunlight than their laptop screen sees them.

3. Clothing practices: Traditional and religious clothing often covers most of the body. Studies show you need to expose at least 40% of your body surface area for more than 30 minutes daily to maintain normal vitamin D status. That's not happening when you're wrapped in layers in the name of modesty or fashion.

4. Air pollution: Remember that pollution blanket we discussed? It filters out UVB radiation too. Living in Delhi during winter means you're getting sunlight that's been filtered through what essentially amounts to an atmospheric cigarette.

5. Sunscreen obsession: Here's where dermatologists and endocrinologists have a polite disagreement. Dermatologists rightfully warn about skin cancer and photoaging. Endocrinologists point to the vitamin D crisis. The truth? Most sunscreens don't block enough UVB to completely prevent vitamin D synthesis, but consistent use does reduce it. The solution isn't ditching sunscreen—it's about smart, brief exposure and dietary supplementation.

Melanin: Your Built-In Sunscreen (That Still Needs Backup)

Indian skin typically has higher levels of eumelanin, the type of melanin that provides better UV protection compared to lighter skin tones. This is why non-melanoma skin cancers are relatively less common in India compared to Western countries—our Age-Standardized Rates are much lower.

But—and this is a crucial but—melanin protection is not absolute. It's more like having a shield with a few holes in it rather than no shield at all. UV radiation still causes DNA damage in all skin types. Melanin reduces risk; it doesn't eliminate it. Skin cancer rates are climbing in India, particularly in urban areas with better diagnostic access. A study analyzing cancer registry data found significant regional variation: northeastern regions showed higher incidence due to increased UV exposure, while regions along the Ganges basin showed higher rates potentially linked to arsenic exposure.

The lesson? Don't let the melanin lull you into false security. Protection matters regardless of skin tone.

The Brain Chemistry Connection: Serotonin, Dopamine, and Why You Feel Better After a Walk

Sunlight does more than just synthesize vitamins and tan your skin—it fundamentally affects your brain chemistry. When sunlight enters your eyes (no, you don't have to stare at the Sun like some overzealous yoga guru), it hits special photosensitive cells in your retina. These cells contain melanopsin, a photopigment that's particularly sensitive to blue light around 477 nanometers.

These cells communicate directly with the suprachiasmatic nucleus (SCN) in your hypothalamus—essentially your brain's master clock. This triggers several cascading effects:

Serotonin regulation: Bright light exposure increases serotonin production in the brain. Serotonin is your brain's mood stabilizer, affecting everything from happiness to focus. Low serotonin levels are associated with depression, including Seasonal Affective Disorder (SAD). This is why you feel notably better after a morning walk than after doom-scrolling in bed—one involves sunlight-triggered serotonin, the other involves Twitter-triggered cortisol.

Melatonin suppression during the day: Sunlight suppresses melatonin, the sleep hormone, keeping you alert during daytime. When evening arrives and light diminishes, melatonin production ramps up, preparing you for sleep. This is your circadian rhythm in action.

Dopamine effects: Recent research suggests UV exposure can increase dopamine levels in the brain and peripheral organs. While we often associate dopamine with reward and pleasure, it also affects memory formation and neurogenesis. Interestingly, excessive UV exposure may lead to memory deficits through dopamine dysregulation, which is nature's way of saying everything in moderation, including sunbathing.

Studies show that morning sunlight exposure is particularly crucial for good sleep that night. Even 30 minutes of morning sunlight helps regulate your circadian rhythm, advancing your clock so you feel sleepy earlier and wake up refreshed. Evening sunlight has the opposite effect—it delays your clock, making you sleep and wake later. This explains why working night shifts or pulling all-nighters for that IIT-JEE prep feels so biologically wrong—because it is.

Seasonal Affective Disorder: Winter Blues, Indian Edition

"But we're in India, we have sunshine all year, SAD doesn't affect us, right?"

Wrong. While SAD is less prevalent in tropical countries than in Scandinavia (where winter means three hours of daylight and existential dread), it does occur in India. The lack of sufficient sunlight during shorter winter days can disrupt circadian rhythms and decrease serotonin levels, leading to persistent low mood, low energy, oversleeping, carbohydrate cravings, and social withdrawal.

Interestingly, summer-pattern SAD—less common but equally valid—also occurs, particularly in India and Pakistan where extreme heat may trigger symptoms. Light therapy, using devices that emit 10,000 lux of light (about 20 times brighter than typical indoor lighting), has proven effective in treating SAD. Think of it as concentrated, scheduled sunshine without the UV damage—medical science's way of gaming the system.

Real-World Applications in the Indian Context

Solar Energy: Powering India's Tomorrow (If We Stop Polluting Our Skies)

India's solar journey reads like a startup success story. From a mere 2.5 GW installed capacity in 2014 to over 127 GW by September 2025, we've seen a 30-fold surge in adoption. Solar power now constitutes 47% of India's renewable energy capacity, and we're gunning for 500 GW of renewable energy by 2030, with solar expected to contribute at least 250 GW.

The Bhadla Solar Park in Rajasthan generates 2,245 MW—enough to power millions of homes. The Omkareshwar Floating Solar Park in Madhya Pradesh, with its planned 600 MW capacity, showcases innovation: solar panels on water save land and operate more efficiently due to the cooling effect.

Programs like PM Surya Ghar Yojana and PM Kusum Yojana are democratizing solar access, helping households and farmers transition to clean energy. The PM JANMAN scheme aims to electrify one lakh un-electrified tribal households with solar power, addressing energy poverty in remote areas.

But here's the uncomfortable truth: climate change and air pollution threaten to undermine these gains. Research projects that by mid-century (2041-2050), photovoltaic efficiency could decrease by 3.3% due to rising temperatures and increased aerosol pollution. Higher emission scenarios predict solar radiation reductions exceeding 10% by 2100 in key solar regions. Translation: we're building solar infrastructure while simultaneously sabotaging the resource it depends on. It's like opening a seafood restaurant on a dying coral reef.

The solution? Aggressive pollution control, cleaner fuels, and hybrid renewable systems that don't put all eggs in one basket.

Agriculture: Where Sunlight Meets Survival

In a country where agriculture employs about 42% of the workforce, understanding sunlight isn't academic—it's existential. Photosynthesis, the process by which plants convert sunlight into chemical energy, operates at 1-2% efficiency for most plants. C3 plants (wheat, rice, cotton) max out at about 4.6% efficiency, while C4 plants (sugarcane, corn, sorghum) can hit 6% under optimal conditions.

These numbers might seem low compared to commercial solar panels (15-20% efficiency), but plants optimize for survival and reproduction, not pure energy conversion. They need to balance energy capture with water retention, temperature regulation, and defense mechanisms—challenges solar panels don't face.

But declining sunshine hours threaten crop yields. Less sunlight means less photosynthesis means less food production, in a country projected to have 1.5 billion mouths to feed. The aerosol dimming effect isn't just about solar panels—it's about rice yields in Punjab and wheat harvests in Madhya Pradesh.

Agrivoltaics—installing solar panels in agricultural fields in ways that allow farming underneath—presents an innovative solution. Projects in Delhi and Jodhpur demonstrate that you can grow crops and generate electricity on the same land. It's the agricultural equivalent of having your cake and eating it too, assuming the cake generates clean energy.

Circadian Health in the Age of Screens

Modern urban life has created a bizarre situation: we're simultaneously starved for natural daylight and drowning in artificial light. The average person spends over seven hours daily staring at screens, exposing their eyes to blue light (400-500 nm) that suppresses melatonin production and disrupts sleep.

Digital eye strain, characterized by blurred vision, headaches, dry eyes, and neck pain, affects millions. The 20-20-20 rule—every 20 minutes, look at something 20 feet away for 20 seconds—isn't just ergonomic advice; it's physiological necessity.

But here's the paradox: we need blue light exposure during the day for alertness and mood regulation, but it's terrible for us at night. The solution isn't to avoid screens entirely (good luck with that in 2025), but to be strategic: get morning sunlight, use blue light filters on devices in the evening, and for the love of your circadian rhythm, stop scrolling Instagram at 2 AM.

Light Therapy: Medicine Meets Photons

Light therapy has evolved from treating jaundice in newborns (blue light breaks down bilirubin) to addressing a range of conditions:

- Red light therapy (630-850 nm) stimulates cellular healing, reduces inflammation, and is used for wound healing, chronic pain, acne, wrinkles, and even cognitive enhancement.

- Blue light therapy targets acne-causing bacteria on skin surfaces.
- UV phototherapy treats psoriasis and atopic dermatitis under controlled medical settings.
- Bright light therapy (10,000 lux) treats Seasonal Affective Disorder and circadian rhythm disorders.

These aren't wellness fads peddled by influencers—they're evidence-based medical interventions with peer-reviewed research backing. The key is proper application under medical guidance, not DIY experimentation with sketchy devices from shady online marketplaces.

Critical Analysis: Debunking Solar Myths and WhatsApp Science

Myth 1: "Base Tan Protects You From Sunburn"

This myth refuses to die, probably because it sounds logical and gives people an excuse to tan. The truth? A "base tan" provides an SPF of approximately 3 or less, which is essentially useless against actual UV exposure. Any tan—whether from the sun or tanning beds—is evidence of DNA damage to skin cells. You're not building protection; you're accumulating damage. Using tanning beds to "prepare" for vacation is like punching yourself in the face to prepare for a boxing match. It's not strategy; it's just more injury.

Myth 2: "Tanning Beds Are Safer Than Sun Exposure"

Categorically false. One visit to a tanning salon significantly increases melanoma risk. A study of 63 women diagnosed with melanoma before age 30 found that 61 (97%) had used tanning beds. Tanning beds primarily emit UVA radiation, which penetrates deeper and is strongly linked to melanoma. The tanning industry marketed UVA as safer because it doesn't cause immediate sunburn—but that's like marketing arsenic as safe because it doesn't cause immediate stomach pain.

Myth 3: "You Need Unprotected Sun Exposure for Adequate Vitamin D"

This is where things get nuanced. While it's true that UVB exposure synthesizes vitamin D, you don't need prolonged, unprotected exposure. Most people get sufficient vitamin D from:

- Brief incidental exposure: A few minutes daily on face and hands often suffices.
- Dietary sources: Fortified milk, fatty fish, egg yolks, mushrooms.
- Supplements: 600-800 IU daily covers most people's needs.

Even the strongest sunscreens don't block 100% of UVB rays. The skin cancer risk from chronic UV exposure far outweighs any potential vitamin D benefit from tanning. If you're deficient, take a supplement. Don't sacrifice your DNA integrity for marginally better vitamin D synthesis.

Myth 4: "Dark Skin Doesn't Need Sunscreen"

The melanin argument again. Yes, melanin provides some protection—but not immunity. UV radiation causes damage across all skin types, though manifestation differs. Indians may not burn as easily as Caucasians, but photoaging, hyperpigmentation disorders, and yes, skin cancer still occur. The incidence may be lower, but the severity when it occurs can be equal or worse due to late detection.

Myth 5: "Pollution Doesn't Affect How Much Sunlight I Get"

Oh, how wrong this is. Air pollution, particularly PM2.5 and aerosols, significantly reduces surface solar radiation. India's "solar dimming" phenomenon shows sunshine hours declining despite no change in the Sun's output. Those hazy winter skies in Delhi? They're filtering out sunlight, including UVB needed for vitamin D synthesis. You're getting light, but less of the beneficial wavelengths. It's like trying to charge your phone through a dirty screen protector—technically working, but inefficiently.

The Government Policy Critique

India's solar ambitions are admirable—500 GW renewable capacity by 2030 is ambitious and necessary. But policy often ignores the elephant in the room: air quality. You can't achieve optimal solar energy generation with polluted skies. It's like trying to fill a leaky bucket while ignoring the leak.

The National Clean Air Programme exists but lacks teeth in enforcement. Cities routinely breach air quality standards, yet penalties remain minimal and monitoring inadequate. Meanwhile, we're installing solar panels that will operate at reduced efficiency because we haven't addressed the atmospheric pollution causing the dimming.

Similarly, vitamin D deficiency is a recognized public health crisis, yet public health campaigns emphasizing supplementation and dietary sources remain limited. We're great at identifying problems, less great at implementing solutions.

The Scientific Thought Experiment: Imagine India Without Its Sun Tax

Here's a mental exercise: Imagine if India could reduce its air pollution to developed nation levels while maintaining its tropical location. How would life change?

Energy: Solar panels operate at peak efficiency. That 127 GW installed capacity might generate 12-41% more power just from cleaner air. Energy costs drop, grid stability improves, and the 500 GW target becomes more achievable.

Health: Vitamin D levels normalize as UVB reaches the ground unfiltered. Depression rates potentially decline as more people get adequate sunlight exposure for serotonin regulation. Respiratory diseases from PM2.5 decrease, reducing healthcare burden.

Agriculture: Crop yields increase with consistent, unfiltered sunlight for photosynthesis. India's food security strengthens without needing more land or water—just cleaner skies.

Urban planning: People naturally spend more time outdoors when visibility is good and air is breathable. Parks become usable year-round, not just post-monsoon. The mental health benefits compound.

This isn't fantasy—it's achievable with political will, stringent enforcement, and industrial accountability. The question isn't whether we can do it, but whether we're willing to prioritize long-term gains over short-term economic convenience.

The Home Experiment: Track Your Sunlight Exposure

Want to understand your personal relationship with sunlight? Try this two-week experiment:

Week 1 - Track your baseline:

- Note how many hours you spend outdoors in natural light daily.
- Record your energy levels, mood, and sleep quality (1-10 scale).
- Take a vitamin D blood test (optional but informative).

Week 2 - Intervention:

- Get 30 minutes of outdoor sunlight exposure within 2 hours of waking (face and arms exposed).
- Reduce screen time after sunset by 50%.
- Use orange-tinted glasses or screen filters if screens are necessary.
- Continue tracking energy, mood, and sleep quality.

Compare: Most people report improved sleep quality, better morning alertness, and more stable mood. It's not magic—it's just biology working as evolution designed.

The beauty of this experiment? Zero cost, minimal time investment, and tangible benefits you can measure subjectively.

Synthesis: What Does Sunlight Mean for India's Future?

As we stand in 2025, sunlight represents both opportunity and challenge for India. On one hand, our tropical location gives us a natural advantage in solar energy generation—a clean, abundant resource that could power our development aspirations sustainably. On the other hand, our air quality crisis threatens to squander this advantage, literally dimming our skies and reducing the very resource we're trying to harness.

The vitamin D paradox—widespread deficiency in a sun-drenched nation—reflects our disconnect from natural environments and the triumph of cultural preferences (fairness) and modern lifestyles (indoor work) over biological needs. It's a first-world problem in a developing country context: we have the resource, we're just not using it properly.

But perhaps most importantly, sunlight represents a daily reminder of our interconnectedness with natural systems. The same photons that power photosynthesis in rice paddies also regulate your sleep cycle and synthesize vitamins in your skin. The same aerosol pollution that reduces solar panel efficiency also increases your risk of respiratory disease and mood disorders. You can't optimize one part of the system while ignoring others.

For young Indians reading this—the engineering students, the IT professionals, the content creators, the changemakers—understanding sunlight isn't just about acing a physics exam or optimizing vitamin D levels. It's about recognizing that some of the most elegant solutions to modern problems might involve reconnecting with fundamental natural processes we've spent the last century trying to insulate ourselves from.

Practical Takeaways for Your 2025 Life:

1. Get morning sunlight religiously - 20-30 minutes within 2 hours of waking, outdoors if possible. Your circadian rhythm will thank you with better sleep.

2. Use sunscreen intelligently - SPF 30 or higher for prolonged exposure, but don't avoid the sun completely. Brief exposure without sunscreen (10-15 minutes, midday, face and arms) is generally safe for vitamin D.

3. Supplement vitamin D - 600-800 IU daily, more if deficient. Blood test first, supplement second, sunscreen always.

4. Manage screen time strategically - Blue light exposure in the morning: good. Blue light at midnight: terrible for sleep. Orange-tinted glasses or filters for evening screen use.

5. Support clean air initiatives - Your vote matters. Politicians who prioritize air quality are investing in everything from solar efficiency to public health to agricultural productivity.

6. Think generationally - The choices we make about air quality, urban planning, and energy policy today determine whether future Indians will enjoy the same sunshine intensity our grandparents did, or inherit increasingly dimmed skies.

The Final Word (Or: Why Should You Care About Photons?)

Sunlight is simultaneously the most ordinary and most extraordinary thing about Earth. Ordinary because it shows up reliably (pollution notwithstanding), extraordinary because it powers nearly everything living on this planet and influences everything from your mood to your grocery bill.

Understanding sunlight—its physics, its chemistry, its biological effects—isn't pedantic scientific gatekeeping. It's practical knowledge for navigating modern life. It explains why you feel like garbage after a weekend of indoor gaming, why those evening scrolling sessions wreck your sleep, why your grandmother's insistence on morning walks wasn't just tradition but practical wisdom encoded across generations.

It also explains why India's future—energetically, agriculturally, economically—depends partly on maintaining and improving the quality of sunlight reaching our surfaces. We're in a race between our clean energy ambitions and our air pollution trajectory. Which trend wins will determine whether 2050 India is powered by efficient solar grids or by increasingly desperate attempts to squeeze energy from diminishing sunlight.

The Sun will keep shining for another 5 billion years. The question is whether we'll clean up our act in the next 5 years to actually benefit from it.

Now go outside, face east, and let some photons hit your retina. Your circadian rhythm has been waiting patiently for you to finish reading this chapter.

Chapter 2: Fresh Air (PRANA)

The Great Indian Breathing Paradox (Or: How We're Suffocating While Standing Outside)

It's 7 AM in Delhi, and you've just stepped onto your balcony for your morning "fresh air"—quotation marks doing more heavy lifting than your lungs will manage today. The AQI app on your phone cheerfully informs you that the air quality is "Very Poor" at 312, which in normal-people terminology means you're basically vaping a cocktail of vehicular emissions, construction dust, and last month's crop stubble smoke from Punjab. Your fitness app pings a reminder: "Don't forget your morning jog!" Sure, let me just go run through what's essentially an open-air gas chamber. What could go wrong?

Meanwhile, your yoga instructor's Instagram story from yesterday shows them in *padmasana*, captioned: "Breathe in the universe's energy. Prana is free, unlimited, and everywhere." Technically true, if by "everywhere" they mean "trapped under a layer of PM2.5 so thick NASA satellites can see it from space." Welcome to India in 2025, where the ancient concept of *prana*—the vital life force carried by breath—meets the modern reality that the air carrying said life force might also be carrying enough pollutants to age your lungs by a decade.

Here's the kicker: India is home to 6 of the world's 10 most polluted cities, and 13 of the top 20. Delhi remains the world's most polluted capital with PM2.5 concentrations of 91.6 μg/m³, which is roughly 18 times the WHO's recommended safe limit of 5 μg/m³. The country's average PM2.5 level is 50.6 μg/m³—still 10 times above WHO guidelines. And yet, breathing is free, unlimited, and non-negotiable. It's like being told you have unlimited access to a buffet, but 70% of the dishes might slowly poison you. Fun times.

The Science of Breathing (Or: Your Lungs Are Basically Uber For Oxygen)

Let's talk about what breathing actually does, beyond keeping you alive and giving you something to do between Instagram scrolls. Every breath you take (cue The Police) initiates a remarkably elegant molecular delivery system that makes Amazon's same-day delivery look amateur.

The Atmospheric Recipe We're Working With

First, what exactly are you breathing? Earth's atmosphere—when not contaminated by human activities—has a surprisingly consistent composition that's been stable for millions of years:

- 78.08% Nitrogen (N_2) - The filler content of air, chemically inert, mostly just along for the ride
- 20.95% Oxygen (O_2) - The star of the show, the molecule your cells are desperately waiting for
- 0.93% Argon (Ar) - Another noble gas that does basically nothing but take up space
- 0.04% Carbon Dioxide (CO_2) - Tiny percentage, massive importance for regulating your breathing
- Variable Water Vapor (H_2O) - Can be 0-3% depending on humidity
- Trace gases - Neon, helium, methane, and in Indian cities, a generous helping of nitrogen dioxide, sulfur dioxide, and particulate matter not listed in the original atmospheric recipe

Here's the part your 10th-grade biology teacher glossed over: you're not actually using most of what you breathe. Nitrogen passes through your lungs unchanged—it's the ultimate freeloader. What your body is desperately after is that 21% oxygen, which powers the cellular respiration process that keeps every cell in your body functioning.

The Oxygen Delivery System: A Journey

When you inhale, here's the incredible journey each oxygen molecule takes:

1. Entry Point: Air rushes through your nose or mouth (nose is better—it filters, warms, and humidifies the air). Your sinuses act as a temperature regulation system, ensuring air doesn't hit your lungs too cold or too dry.

2. The Highway: Air travels down your trachea, branches into bronchi, then into smaller bronchioles—like a road network going from highway to street to narrow lane. Think of it as Bangalore traffic in reverse: starts wide, gets narrower, but somehow things still flow.

3. The Destination: Air reaches the alveoli—tiny air sacs in your lungs, about 300 million of them, with a total surface area of 70 square meters. If you could spread them out flat, they'd cover roughly half a badminton court. Evolution really went all-in on surface area here.

4. The Exchange: Oxygen diffuses across the alveolar-capillary membrane into your bloodstream. This happens via simple diffusion—no active transport needed, just molecules moving from high concentration to low concentration. Elegant, efficient, and completely automatic.

5. The Taxi Service: Oxygen dissolves into blood plasma, but most of it (about 98.5%) immediately hitches a ride with hemoglobin inside red blood cells. Each hemoglobin molecule can carry four oxygen molecules. It's like a molecular carpooling system.

6. Final Delivery: Oxygen-rich blood travels through arteries to tissues throughout your body. At the destination, a fascinating exchange occurs: cells release carbon dioxide (metabolic waste) while picking up oxygen. The hemoglobin taxi drops off oxygen and picks up CO_2 for the return trip.

This entire process—from inhalation to cellular delivery—happens automatically, about 20,000 times a day. You're running the world's most efficient logistics operation without even thinking about it.

Carbon Dioxide: The Underrated Regulator

Here's where it gets interesting. While oxygen gets all the glory, carbon dioxide is actually what controls your breathing. Your brain doesn't primarily monitor oxygen levels—it monitors CO_2.

When CO_2 levels rise in your blood, it combines with water to form carbonic acid (H_2CO_3), which dissociates into hydrogen ions (H^+) and bicarbonate (HCO_3^-):

$$CO_2 + H_2O \rightleftharpoons H_2CO_3 \rightleftharpoons H^+ + HCO_3^-$$

This is the bicarbonate buffer system, one of your body's primary pH regulation mechanisms. When CO_2 rises, pH drops (becomes more acidic). Chemoreceptors in your brain and carotid arteries detect this pH change and send urgent messages: "Breathe faster, dude!"

This is why when you hold your breath, the burning sensation isn't from lack of oxygen (initially)—it's from CO_2 buildup creating an acidic environment in your blood. It's also why hyperventilation (breathing too fast) makes you feel lightheaded: you're expelling CO_2 too quickly, raising blood pH into alkalotic territory.

The Bohr effect adds another layer of elegance: when CO_2 and H^+ concentrations are high in tissues (where cells are actively working), hemoglobin's affinity for oxygen *decreases*, causing it to release oxygen more readily. Conversely, in the lungs where CO_2 is low, hemoglobin binds oxygen more tightly. It's a self-regulating system that delivers oxygen precisely where it's needed most.

The Indian Respiratory Crisis (Or: When Free Air Comes With Hidden Costs)

Now let's address the elephant in the room—or rather, the PM2.5 in the atmosphere. India's air quality situation has gone from bad to "maybe we should all just move to the Himalayas."

The Numbers Don't Lie (But They Do Hurt)

- India's average PM2.5 level: 50.6 μg/m^3 (2024)
- WHO recommended limit: 5 μg/m^3
- India's national standard: 40 μg/m^3 annual average
- Delhi's PM2.5: 91.6 μg/m^3
- Byrnihat (Assam-Meghalaya border): 128.2 μg/m^3—the most

polluted city in India

Here's the brutal math: Every 10 μg/m³ increase in PM2.5 concentration leads to an 8.6% increase in mortality. India's air pollution caused approximately 1.5 million deaths annually between 2009-2019. Over that decade, 3.8 million deaths were linked to air pollution above India's own lax standards; compared to WHO guidelines, the figure jumps to 16.6 million deaths—almost 25% of all mortality during that period.

To put this in perspective: air pollution kills more Indians annually than COVID-19 did during its worst year. The economic cost? $36.8 billion annually, or 1.36% of GDP. That's not just a public health crisis—it's an economic disaster.

Respiratory Diseases: The Statistics That Should Scare You

India has an estimated 55.3 million people with COPD (Chronic Obstructive Pulmonary Disease) and 37.9 million with asthma as of 2016. COPD prevalence is 4.2%, asthma is 2.9%. The burden of chronic respiratory diseases has increased from 4.5% of total DALYs (Disability-Adjusted Life Years) in 1990 to 6.4% in 2016. Of the total global burden of chronic respiratory diseases, 32% occurs in India despite having only 18% of the world's population.

Here's the painful part: the DALYs per person with COPD or asthma are 1.7 and 2.4 times higher in India than the global average. Translation: Indians with these conditions suffer more and die earlier than their counterparts elsewhere, primarily due to late diagnosis, poor management, and continued exposure to pollutants.

The leading risk factors for COPD in India:

- 53.7% attributable to air pollution (both ambient and household)
- 25.4% to tobacco use
- 16.5% to occupational risks

Notably, air pollution is the *dominant* risk factor—outpacing even tobacco, unlike in Western countries where smoking leads. This is because of India's unique challenge: high ambient air pollution *plus* widespread use of biomass fuels for cooking in rural areas.

Indoor Air Pollution: The Invisible Killer

Here's a fun fact that'll ruin your day: indoor air can be 2-5 times more polluted than outdoor air. A study of 30 office spaces across nine Indian cities found that 73% were non-compliant with indoor air quality limits. In 67% of offices, nitrogen dioxide levels exceeded recommended thresholds.

Sources of indoor air pollution:

- Cooking: Deep frying, gas stoves, and biomass burning release PM2.5, volatile organic compounds (VOCs), nitrogen oxides (NO_x), and carbon monoxide
- Cleaning products: Sprays, disinfectants, air fresheners release VOCs
- Building materials: Paint, furniture, carpets off-gas formaldehyde and other chemicals
- Infiltration: Outdoor pollution seeps indoors through doors, windows, and ventilation

In Delhi-NCR, even with closed doors, naturally ventilated buildings showed CO_2 levels reaching 3,900 ppm—well above the 1,000 ppm recommended limit. The cruel irony: keeping windows closed to avoid outdoor pollution traps indoor pollutants, and opening them invites the outdoor smog inside. It's a lose-lose situation.

A study found that 56.8% of participants reported one or more symptoms related to air pollution, with eye irritation (30%) and respiratory issues (23%) being most common. Indoor air pollution contributes significantly to the 70% of Kolkata residents suffering from respiratory diseases.

Pranayama and Breathwork (Or: Ancient Wisdom Meets Modern Science)

Now, let's talk about *pranayama*—the millennia-old yogic breathing practices that your grandmother swears by and your dermatologist doesn't understand. Turns out, both ancient yogis and modern scientists agree: how you breathe matters almost as much as what you breathe.

The Science Behind Conscious Breathing

A systematic review of controlled trials found that pranayama significantly improves:

- Cardiorespiratory function: Pulse rate, systolic blood pressure, forced vital capacity (FVC), forced expiratory volume (FEV_1), and peak expiratory flow rate (PEFR) all improved
- Asthma symptoms: Reduced frequency of attacks, severity, and medication requirements; improved quality of life
- COPD symptoms: Better symptom scores, activity levels, and impact scores
- Cardiovascular health: Reduced heart rate, blood pressure, and anxiety in cardiac patients
- Mental health: Improved emotions, reduced fatigue, better sleep, decreased anxiety in cancer patients

The mechanisms are multifaceted:

1. Mechanical Effects: Deep, controlled breathing exercises respiratory muscles—both inspiratory and expiratory. Techniques like *Bhastrika* (bellows breath) and *Kapalbhati* (skull-shining breath) strengthen the diaphragm and abdominal muscles, improving overall lung capacity. Deep inspiration near total lung capacity stimulates surfactant release, increasing lung compliance.

2. Airway Effects: Slow, gentle breathing reduces frictional stress in airways, stabilizing mast cell degranulation and reducing inflammation and airway obstruction. This is particularly beneficial for asthma patients.

3. Autonomic Regulation: This is where it gets fascinating. Pranayama shifts the autonomic nervous system balance from sympathetic (fight-or-flight) to parasympathetic (rest-and-digest) dominance. Slow breathing generates inhibitory signals and hyperpolarizing currents that synchronize neural elements, promoting relaxation.

Vagal afferents from lung stretch receptors connect to the nucleus tractus solitarius, which sends fibers to the thalamus, limbic areas, and anterior cortical areas. This is the physiological basis for why controlled breathing calms your mind—it's literally a neural circuit connecting your lungs to your emotional centers.

4. Neurochemical Effects: Pranayama increases melatonin production,

promoting relaxation and well-being. Breath-holding induces theta waves in EEG, associated with meditative states. Some research suggests pranayama can modulate dopamine and serotonin levels, though the mechanisms are still being studied.

Breathwork for Mental Health

Modern research confirms what yogis knew: breathwork is powerful medicine for the mind. Studies show that even simple breathing techniques reduce stress, anxiety, and depression.

A meta-analysis found breathwork interventions were associated with significant reductions in:

- Stress: Effect size of -0.35 (small to medium improvement)
- Anxiety: Effect size of -0.32
- Depression: Effect size of -0.40

Particularly effective was cyclic sighing—slow inhalation followed by extended exhalation. Participants practicing this for just 5 minutes daily experienced greater improvements in positive affect than those doing mindfulness meditation. The daily increase in positive feelings was about one-third greater than the meditation group.

Why does it work? Controlled breathing activates the parasympathetic nervous system, triggering the relaxation response. Deep breathing signals to your brain that it's safe to calm down. When you exhale slowly, you're literally hacking your nervous system to chill out.

The 4-7-8 technique (inhale for 4 seconds, hold for 7, exhale for 8) is particularly effective for anxiety and insomnia. Box breathing (4 counts each for inhale, hold, exhale, hold) is used by Navy SEALs to maintain calm under pressure. These aren't woo-woo wellness trends—they're evidence-based interventions with measurable physiological effects.

Real-World Applications and Solutions

The Air Purifier Reality Check

Given India's air quality, air purifiers have become as common as pressure cookers in urban homes. But do they actually work?

Yes, but (there's always a but).

HEPA (High-Efficiency Particulate Air) filters capture 99.97% of particles ≥0.3 microns. Studies in India found HEPA purifiers reduced indoor PM levels by:

- 12-52% in general indoor air (Air Purifier I)
- 37-64% in general indoor air (Air Purifier II)
- 29-53% with external pollution sources like candles/incense (Air Purifier I)
- 52-68% with external pollution sources (Air Purifier II)

Another study found air filters reduced indoor fine particle concentrations by 60% and increased reactive hyperemia (a measure of vascular function) by 9.4%.

The catch:

- HEPA filters trap particles but not gases like nitrogen dioxide, ozone, or VOCs. You need activated carbon filters for those.
- Many cheap devices labeled "HEPA-type" or "HEPA-like" don't meet the 99.97% efficiency standard. They're essentially expensive fans.
- One purifier won't protect your entire home. They work locally—the room they're in. Thinking one living room unit protects your bedroom is wishful thinking.
- CADR (Clean Air Delivery Rate) matters. A purifier must have appropriate CADR for room size to achieve multiple air changes per hour.
- Filters need replacement every 6-12 months at ₹2,000-5,000 per filter. Budget accordingly.
- Running them continuously is crucial. Pollutants re-accumulate quickly when off.

Bottom line: HEPA purifiers are effective tools but not magic shields. They're one component of a comprehensive strategy that should include source control (reducing indoor pollution), proper ventilation when outdoor AQI permits, and policy-level changes to ambient air quality.

Forest Bathing: Nature's Air Purification

Here's a delightful piece of science that sounds like it came from a wellness influencer but is actually peer-reviewed: spending time in forests measurably boosts your immune system.

The secret? Phytoncides—volatile organic compounds released by trees, especially conifers. When inhaled, these compounds:

- Increase natural killer (NK) cell activity by up to 50%, lasting for 7-30 days after a forest visit
- Increase anti-cancer proteins (perforin, granzymes, granulysin) in immune cells
- Reduce cortisol, adrenaline, and blood pressure
- Improve mood and reduce anxiety
- Enhance focus and reduce cognitive fatigue

The effect is specific to forests—city park visits don't produce the same immune boost. Alpha-pinene and beta-pinene, detected in forest air but nearly absent in cities, appear to be key active compounds.

A forest bathing trip doesn't mean hiking—it's about slow, mindful presence. Walk slowly, sit frequently, engage all senses. The Japanese practice of *shinrin-yoku* (forest bathing) is now prescribed by doctors as preventive medicine.

For urban Indians with limited forest access, even small green spaces help. Parks with mature trees, botanical gardens, or urban forests provide benefits. The key is spending time among trees, breathing deeply, and disconnecting from digital noise.

Critical Analysis: Myths, Misconceptions, and WhatsApp Science

Myth 1: "Deep breathing exercises cure respiratory diseases"

No. Let's be clear: pranayama and breathwork are complementary therapies, not replacements for medical treatment. They improve symptoms, reduce medication requirements, and enhance quality of life in asthma and COPD patients, but they don't cure the diseases.

If you have COPD or asthma, keep using your inhalers. Add pranayama, don't substitute it. There's even a reported case of pneumothorax (collapsed lung) from aggressive *Kapalbhati* practice in someone with compromised lungs. Practice under supervision if you have respiratory conditions.

Myth 2: "Morning air is the purest"

Depends on where you live. In cities, early morning can actually have *higher* pollution due to the atmospheric inversion layer—cold air traps pollutants close to the ground. Vehicle emissions from early commuters accumulate. The best time for outdoor activity is mid-morning to early afternoon when the atmosphere has mixed and dispersed pollutants—assuming AQI permits outdoor exercise at all.

Rural areas are different. Morning air is genuinely fresher there, assuming no nearby crop burning or industrial sources.

Myth 3: "Air purifiers with ionizers are better"

Actually, avoid ionizers. They can generate ozone as a byproduct, which is a respiratory irritant and can worsen asthma. Stick to mechanical HEPA filtration. Simplicity wins.

Myth 4: "Houseplants significantly purify indoor air"

The beloved NASA study on air-purifying plants used sealed chambers with single plants and measured over extended periods. In real homes with normal ventilation, you'd need 10-1,000 plants per square meter to achieve meaningful air purification. Your money is better spent on a good HEPA filter.

Plants are great for aesthetics, mental health, and minor humidity regulation—just don't expect them to tackle Delhi's smog.

Myth 5: "India's air quality standards are protective"

India's annual PM2.5 standard of 40 $\mu g/m^3$ is 8 times higher than WHO's 5 $\mu g/m^3$ guideline. Research shows even air within India's "safe" limits causes significant mortality. A study found 33,000 annual deaths in 10 cities from air marked safe by Indian standards.

Current standards were set in 2009 before extensive health evidence emerged. They need urgent revision. Relying on government standards for "safe" air is like trusting BMC to tell you when streets will flood—they're consistently optimistic.

The Policy Critique

India's National Clean Air Programme (NCAP), launched in 2019, aims for 20-30% reduction in PM2.5 and PM10 by 2024. Good goal. Execution? Patchy. Only 101 of 131 non-attainment cities under NCAP have functioning continuous air quality monitoring systems. You can't manage what you don't measure.

The Graded Response Action Plan (GRAP) for Delhi-NCR only kicks in during "severe" episodes. But research shows even "moderate" air quality increases mortality. We need year-round action, not crisis management.

The elephant in the policy room: enforcement. Penalties for violating emissions standards remain minimal. Industrial lobbies resist stricter regulations. Stubble burning continues despite bans because farmers lack viable alternatives. Vehicle emission standards exist on paper; implementation is theatrical at best.

Without political will, monitoring infrastructure, and enforcement, policies are feel-good announcements that change little on the ground.

The Thought Experiment: Breathing as a Human Right

Here's a radical idea: What if India treated clean air as a fundamental right, like the right to vote or freedom of speech?

Imagine:

- Mandatory real-time AQI displays in all public spaces, schools, offices
- Air quality-based school closures when AQI exceeds safe thresholds, like weather-based closures
- Stricter vehicle emission standards actually enforced through automated monitoring
- Subsidies for biomass alternatives so farmers don't burn stubble
- Green building codes mandating ventilation systems with filtration in new construction
- Public transport expansion reducing vehicular emissions
- Industrial emission limits with real penalties for violations

This isn't fantasy—it's policy. Beijing reduced PM2.5 by 40% between 2013-2017 through aggressive action. If China can do it, why not India?

The cost of inaction: 1.5 million preventable deaths annually. The economic argument alone—$36.8 billion in annual losses—should justify massive investment in air quality. That's more than India spends on many government schemes.

The Home Experiment: Measure What You Breathe

Want to understand your personal exposure? Try this:

Week 1 - Baseline Data:

- Download an AQI monitoring app (AQI.in, AirVisual, or similar)
- Check AQI three times daily: morning, afternoon, evening
- Note when you spend time outdoors
- Track any respiratory symptoms: cough, irritation, wheezing

Week 2 - Intervention:

- Practice 5 minutes of cyclic sighing daily: slow inhale through nose, slow exhale through mouth (exhale twice as long as inhale)
- Use HEPA purifier continuously in one room if available
- Avoid outdoor activity when AQI exceeds 150 (if possible)
- Continue tracking symptoms

Compare: Most people notice subjective improvements in breathing quality and symptom reduction with minimal intervention. You'll also develop awareness of how outdoor AQI correlates with your symptoms—knowledge that informs better decisions.

If you have respiratory conditions, consult your doctor before starting breathwork. Some practices may not suit everyone.

Synthesis: The Future of Breathing in India

We're at an inflection point. India's air quality has worsened over the past three decades despite growing awareness. But change is possible. The 7% reduction in PM2.5 from 2023 to 2024 shows interventions can work when implemented.

For young Indians, the stakes are personal and immediate. You're inheriting both the problem and the responsibility for solving it. Your lungs are aging faster than they should. Your productivity, cognition, and lifespan are all impacted by air quality.

Practical actions for your 2025 life:

1. Monitor and respond: Use AQI apps. Adjust outdoor activities based on real-time data, not assumptions.

2. Create clean air zones: Invest in quality HEPA purifiers for bedrooms and workspaces. You spend 80-90% of your time indoors—make that air count.

3. Practice breathwork daily: 5-10 minutes of pranayama or controlled breathing. It's free, portable, and evidence-based medicine for both body and mind.

4. Reduce personal emissions: Use public transport, carpool, consider electric vehicles. Individual choices aggregate to systemic change.

5. Seek nature exposure: Weekly visits to parks or urban forests. Monthly trips to actual forests if possible. Your immune system will thank you.

6. Advocate for policy change: Vote for leaders prioritizing air quality. Demand enforcement of existing regulations. Support litigation holding polluters accountable.

7. Spread awareness: Share this knowledge. Air pollution thrives on ignorance. Science-literate citizens create political pressure for change.

The Final Word (Or: Why Breathing Shouldn't Be This Complicated)

Prana—the ancient Vedic concept of life force carried by breath—was supposed to be simple, free, and universally accessible. The *Upanishads* speak of prana as the fundamental energy permeating existence, the bridge between physical body and consciousness. They never mentioned you'd need a ₹30,000 air purifier and an AQI app to safely practice pranayama.

But here we are. In 2025 India, accessing clean air requires awareness, resources, and sometimes luck—particularly geographic luck. The irony is thick enough to measure on a particulate matter sensor.

Yet understanding the science of breathing—from the molecular choreography of gas exchange to the neurochemistry of controlled breathing to the environmental determinants of air quality—empowers you. Knowledge converts helplessness into agency, despair into action.

Your lungs are filtering about 11,000 liters of air daily. Every breath is a choice: where, when, how consciously you breathe. Every policy decision about air quality is a collective choice about whose lungs matter. Every ₹100 you spend on a HEPA filter or public transport instead of personal vehicle is a vote for cleaner air.

The science is clear: air pollution is killing 1.5 million Indians annually. The solutions exist: enforcement of emissions standards, transition to clean fuels, expansion of public transport, industrial regulations with teeth. What's missing is political will and public pressure.

So yes, breathe deeply. Practice your pranayama. Buy the air purifier. Take that forest walk. But also vote, advocate, and refuse to accept poisoned air as India's inevitable destiny. Fresh air shouldn't be a luxury good available only to those who can afford filtration systems and weekend escapes to hill stations.

Prana is supposed to be free. Let's make it clean, too.

Now close this chapter, step outside (check the AQI first), and take ten slow, conscious breaths. Notice how your body feels. Notice the quality of air. Notice what needs to change.

And then work to change it.

CHAPTER 3: PURE WATER

The H_2O Hustle (Or: Why Your ₹30,000 RO Purifier Can't Fix Everything)

It's 8 AM in a typical Indian household, and the drama is unfolding. Your mother is lecturing your cousin who just drank tap water directly—*"Do you want to get typhoid? Have you forgotten what happened to Sharma uncle?"* Your father is checking the RO purifier's filter indicator, muttering about the ₹4,500 replacement cost. Meanwhile, your Instagram feed shows an influencer in Goa claiming that "alkaline water with pH 9.5 changed my life" while your WhatsApp family group forwards a message about how "drinking warm water cures everything from diabetes to heartbreak."

Welcome to India 2025, where water—the most abundant molecule in our bodies and the literal foundation of life—has somehow become more complicated than filing your IT returns. We're a nation where 70% of surface water is unfit for consumption, yet we'll happily debate whether room temperature or lukewarm water is "healthier" while ignoring that the water itself might contain enough fluoride to give you skeletal fluorosis.

Here's the absurd math: India has only 4% of the world's freshwater resources despite housing 18% of the global population. We rank 120 out of 122 countries in the water quality index. Twenty-one major cities, including Delhi and Bengaluru, are expected to deplete their groundwater by 2030. Meanwhile, the typical urban Indian spends more time choosing between Bisleri and Kinley than understanding what's actually in their water. It's peak 21st-century irony: drowning in bottled water options while collectively dying of thirst.

The Chemistry of H_2O (Or: Why This Simple Molecule Is Anything But Simple)

Let's start with what should be the easy part: water's molecular structure. H_2O—one oxygen atom covalently bonded to two hydrogen atoms. Simple, right? Your 10th standard chemistry teacher probably said so. Plot twist: water is one of the weirdest, most complex substances on Earth, and its bizarre properties are precisely why life exists.

The Bent Molecule That Changed Everything

Water's molecular geometry is bent, not linear, with an H-O-H bond angle of 104.5° (or 104.45° if you want to impress people at parties). This happens because oxygen has two lone pairs of electrons that repel the O-H bonds, creating that distinctive V-shape.

Why does this matter? Because the bent shape, combined with oxygen's high electronegativity (3.44 on the Pauling scale versus hydrogen's 2.20), creates a polar molecule. The oxygen end becomes partially negative (δ-), and the hydrogen ends become partially positive (δ+). This polarity is the foundation for literally everything water does.

Hydrogen Bonding: The Molecular Velcro

Here's where water gets genuinely weird. The slightly positive hydrogen of one water molecule is attracted to the slightly negative oxygen of another, forming a hydrogen bond. Each water molecule can form up to four hydrogen bonds—two as a donor (from its hydrogens) and two as an acceptor (to its oxygen's lone pairs).

Hydrogen bonds are weaker than covalent bonds (about 5-30 kJ/mol versus 400+ kJ/mol for O-H covalent bonds), but their cumulative effect is massive. They give water:

1. High boiling point: Water boils at 100°C. Compare this to hydrogen sulfide (H_2S), which has similar structure but boils at -60°C because sulfur's lower electronegativity creates weaker hydrogen bonds. If water

followed the pattern of similar molecules, it should boil around -80°C and we'd all be dead.

2. High specific heat capacity: Water can absorb huge amounts of heat energy with minimal temperature change (4.186 J/g·°C). This is why coastal climates are moderate—oceans act as thermal buffers—and why your body's 60% water content prevents you from overheating during that 2 PM Chennai summer walk.

3. High heat of vaporization: It takes 2,260 kJ to evaporate 1 kg of water. This is why sweating works as cooling—when sweat evaporates, it carries away enormous heat energy, keeping you from spontaneously combusting during Bangalore traffic.

4. Cohesion and adhesion: Water molecules stick to each other (cohesion) and to other polar surfaces (adhesion). This is how trees move water from roots to leaves against gravity via capillary action in xylem vessels. It's also why you can fill a glass slightly above the rim—surface tension from hydrogen bonding holds it together.

5. Universal solvent properties: Water's polarity lets it dissolve ions and other polar molecules. Salt (NaCl) dissociates in water because water molecules surround and stabilize Na^+ and Cl^- ions. This is why blood can transport nutrients, why cells function, why basically everything biochemical happens.

6. Density anomaly: Ice is *less dense* than liquid water, which is bizarre. Most substances are denser in solid form. But ice's crystalline structure locks hydrogen bonds in place, creating more space between molecules. This is why ice floats, why lakes freeze from the top down (allowing aquatic life to survive underneath), and why water pipes burst in Shimla winters.

Biological Importance: Water as Life's Operating System

Water isn't just important for biology—it *is* biology. Every single biological process depends on water's properties:

- Enzyme function: Water molecules stabilize enzyme-substrate complexes through hydrogen bonding, lowering activation energy for reactions. Many reactions require water as a direct participant, donating or accepting protons.

- Protein folding: Hydrophobic amino acids cluster inside proteins to avoid water, while hydrophilic ones face outward to interact with water. This hydrophobic effect drives protein tertiary structure. Without water, proteins wouldn't fold correctly, and you'd be a puddle of dysfunctional molecules.
- DNA structure: Hydrogen bonds between complementary base pairs (A-T, G-C) hold the double helix together. Water also forms a hydration shell around DNA, stabilizing its structure.
- Membrane structure: Cell membranes self-assemble because phospholipid tails are hydrophobic and heads are hydrophilic. Water drives this organization.
- Temperature regulation: Your body is 60% water specifically because water's high specific heat buffers temperature changes. Even vigorous exercise raises body temperature slowly because water absorbs heat energy without dramatic temperature increases.

The phrase "water is life" isn't poetic—it's literal biochemistry.

India's Water Crisis: The Numbers That Should Terrify You

Now let's ruin your day with reality. India's water situation is catastrophically bad and getting worse.

Groundwater Contamination: The Invisible Poison

The Annual Groundwater Quality Report 2024 by the Central Ground Water Board assessed 15,259 monitoring locations and found widespread contamination:

- 19.8% of samples exceeded permissible nitrate limits (>45 mg/L)
- 9.04% exceeded fluoride limits (>1.5 mg/L)
- 3.55% exceeded arsenic limits (>10 ppb)
- 13.20% exceeded iron limits
- 6.60% exceeded uranium limits (>30 ppb)
- 7.25% exceeded electrical conductivity limits, indicating salinity issues

Nitrate contamination affects 56% of India's districts, primarily from agricultural runoff and nitrogen-based fertilizers. Rajasthan, Karnataka, Tamil Nadu, Maharashtra, Telangana, Andhra Pradesh, and Madhya

Pradesh show severe contamination, with over 40% of samples exceeding limits in some states. Maharashtra alone has seven of the fifteen most affected districts.

Fluoride contamination affects 263 districts across 27 states. Rajasthan shows levels up to 31 mg/L—over 20 times the safe limit. Long-term exposure causes fluorosis, a condition involving dental discoloration, skeletal deformities, and neurological damage. Over 25 million people across 17 states drink fluoride-contaminated water daily.

Arsenic contamination plagues 230 districts in 25 states, particularly in Ganga and Brahmaputra floodplains—West Bengal, Jharkhand, Bihar, Uttar Pradesh, Assam, Manipur, Punjab, and Chhattisgarh. Chronic arsenic exposure causes skin lesions, cancer, and cardiovascular disease.

Post-monsoon analysis showed nitrate contamination *increased* from 30.77% pre-monsoon to 32.66% post-monsoon, meaning rainfall is washing more agricultural chemicals into aquifers. The monsoon, traditionally seen as a blessing, is now also a contamination delivery system. That's bleak.

The Human Cost: Disease and Death

The health impacts are staggering:

- 37.7 million Indians affected by waterborne diseases annually
- 200,000 deaths per year from contaminated water
- 400,000-500,000 children under five die annually from diarrhea
- 117,000 under-5 children died from diarrhea in 2015 alone—13% of all under-5 deaths
- 73 million working days lost annually due to waterborne diseases
- Economic cost: $600 million per year

In Odisha and West Bengal, 45.2% of urban and 66.1% of rural households in Odisha don't treat water before drinking. In West Bengal, it's worse: 73.5% urban and 93.3% rural households. These numbers aren't just statistics—they're preventable tragedies.

Waterborne diseases include cholera, diarrhea, dysentery, hepatitis A, typhoid, and polio. The reported incidence of viral hepatitis is 12 per 100,000, but studies suggest the real number is closer to 100 per

100,000. Only a small fraction of cases get reported due to poor epidemiological surveillance.

The average cost of illness per household in Odisha and West Bengal is ₹47.69. For lower-income households (Q1 and Q2 quartiles), this represents 24% and 16% of illness cases respectively. When you're earning ₹10,000/month, a waterborne illness isn't just uncomfortable—it's financially catastrophic.

Water Scarcity: Running Dry

The scarcity situation is equally terrifying:

- 26% of India's land area affected by drought in 2024, with 9% experiencing extreme drought
- Karnataka declared 223 out of 236 taluks drought-affected
- 48 lakh hectares of crops lost in Karnataka alone, worth ₹35,162 crore
- Maharashtra extended drought declaration to 66% of administrative areas (1,532 of 2,292 revenue circles)
- Bengaluru: 6,900 out of 13,900 borewells ran dry despite drilling to 1,500 feet

India's annual per capita water availability is 1,486 cubic meters, projected to fall to 1,367 cubic meters by 2031 as population grows. By 2030, water demand will exceed supply by 70%. Moody's Ratings warns that water scarcity could hurt India's sovereign credit strength by disrupting agriculture and industry, potentially causing social unrest.

Only 31% of industrial and domestic sewage from 23 big cities is treated; the rest flows raw into water bodies. India produces 40 million liters of wastewater daily, with 90% discharged untreated. Industries dump 300-400 million tonnes of waste into water annually.

The irony: we're polluting our limited water while simultaneously running out of it. It's like setting your house on fire while complaining about the cold.

Water Purification: What Actually Works (And What's Just Marketing)

Given the contamination reality, let's talk about purification methods—what science says actually works versus what gets peddled by WhatsApp forwards and Instagram wellness influencers.

Boiling Water: The Old Reliable (With Serious Limitations)

Boiling water at 100°C for at least 1-3 minutes kills most bacteria, viruses, and parasites. It's been the go-to emergency purification method for centuries and works well for biological contaminants.

The limitations:

1. Doesn't remove chemical contaminants: Fluoride, arsenic, nitrates, heavy metals, pesticides—boiling doesn't touch them. If anything, it concentrates them as water evaporates.
2. Doesn't remove TDS: Total Dissolved Solids (minerals, salts) remain unchanged. If your water has high TDS (>500 ppm), boiling won't help.
3. Energy intensive: Takes 10+ minutes to boil and cool water. Not sustainable for daily use at scale.
4. Reduces water quantity: Evaporation means less water to drink.
5. Doesn't eliminate all microorganisms: Some heat-resistant spores survive. Boiled water can be re-contaminated during storage, especially in plastic bottles that leach BPA.

Verdict: Boiling is excellent for emergencies and biological contamination in rural areas without purifiers. But it's insufficient for India's multi-pollutant reality.

Reverse Osmosis (RO): The Heavy-Duty Filter

RO systems use pressure (typically 35-70 psi) to push water through a semipermeable membrane with pores around 0.0001 microns. This removes:

- 99.7% of contaminants including dissolved salts, heavy metals, arsenic, fluoride, nitrates, pharmaceuticals, microplastics
- Bacteria, viruses, parasites (pore size is smaller than these organisms)
- TDS reduction from 1,000+ ppm to 50-200 ppm

The advantages:

- Comprehensive purification covering biological and chemical contaminants

- No heat required (unlike boiling)
- Improves taste by removing chlorine and dissolved substances
- Automatic operation—turn on tap, get purified water

The downsides:

- Water wastage: Typical RO systems reject 3-4 liters for every 1 liter purified. That's 75-80% waste.
- Removes beneficial minerals: Calcium, magnesium, potassium get filtered out along with contaminants. Modern systems add minerals back, but cheaper ones don't.
- Expensive: Initial cost ₹8,000-30,000+, annual maintenance ₹5,000-8,000
- Electricity dependent: Won't work during power cuts without backup
- Requires pre-filtration: Sediment filters needed to protect the RO membrane

When you need RO: If your water has high TDS (>500 ppm), heavy metals, fluoride, arsenic, or nitrates—RO is non-negotiable. Given India's groundwater contamination reality, most urban and many rural areas need RO.

UV Purification: The Microbe Assassin

UV systems expose water to ultraviolet light (wavelength 254 nm) that damages microbial DNA, rendering bacteria, viruses, and parasites unable to reproduce. UV purification:

- Kills 99.99% of microorganisms without chemicals
- Doesn't alter taste, odor, or pH
- No water wastage
- Energy-efficient (uses about 40-60 watts)
- Fast—works in seconds as water flows through

The catch:

- Only works on biological contaminants. Doesn't remove chemicals, heavy metals, TDS, fluoride, or nitrates.
- Effectiveness drops in turbid (cloudy) water—particles block UV light.
- Requires pre-filtration for sediment
- Provides no residual disinfection—water can be recontaminated

post-treatment

When you need UV: If your water source has low TDS and chemical contaminants but biological contamination is the concern—municipal tap water in cities with decent infrastructure. Often combined with RO for comprehensive treatment.

The Optimal Home System

For most Indian homes dealing with contaminated groundwater or unreliable municipal supply, a multi-stage system works best:

1. Sediment filter: Removes dirt, rust, suspended particles
2. Activated carbon filter: Removes chlorine, VOCs, improves taste/odor
3. RO membrane: Removes dissolved contaminants, TDS, heavy metals
4. Mineralizer: Adds back calcium, magnesium for health and taste
5. UV chamber: Final disinfection to ensure no microbial survival

Yes, it's expensive. Yes, it wastes water. But given India's water quality, it's also necessary. The alternative is chronic exposure to contaminants that cause cancer, fluorosis, and developmental disorders.

Desalination: The Coastal Solution

India has built multiple seawater desalination plants, particularly in Chennai, which faces chronic water scarcity:

- Minjur Plant (2010): 100 MLD (million liters per day), India's first large-scale plant, serves 2.5 million people
- Nemmeli Plant: 100 MLD
- Perur Plant (under construction, completion 2026): 400 MLD, will be Asia's largest
- Jamnagar Plant (Gujarat): 160 MLD, serving Reliance refinery operations

Desalination uses reverse osmosis to remove salt and minerals from seawater. For every 100 MLD output, plants draw 237 MLD raw seawater. The reject brine (concentrated saltwater) is disposed back into the ocean 650m offshore.

Advantages:

- Coastal areas have unlimited seawater supply
- Eliminates dependence on monsoons, rivers, groundwater
- Better quality control than relying on contaminated freshwater sources
- Costs have decreased—now competitive with long-distance water transport

Challenges:

- Energy-intensive process
- High capital cost (₹500-600 crore for 100 MLD plants)
- Requires coastal location
- Brine disposal has environmental impact on marine ecosystems

Chennai's success demonstrates desalination viability for coastal cities facing scarcity. As water stress intensifies, expect more cities to adopt this approach.

Critical Analysis: Debunking Water Myths and WhatsApp Wisdom

Now let's address the absurd myths circulating in Indian homes, forwarded by your well-meaning but scientifically illiterate relatives.

Myth 1: "Alkaline Water Cures Everything"

The alkaline water trend claims that drinking water with pH 8-9.5 improves hydration, digestion, slows aging, prevents disease, and basically turns you into a superhuman.

The reality: Your body's pH is tightly regulated at 7.35-7.45 by your kidneys and respiratory system. Drinking alkaline water does precisely nothing to your body's pH because your stomach immediately neutralizes it with hydrochloric acid (pH ~1.5-3). The gastric juices bring alkaline water back to acidic before it even enters your intestines.

Any claimed digestive benefits disappear once you understand basic physiology. Your body *needs* stomach acid to digest food and kill pathogens. Neutralizing it with alkaline water isn't helpful—it's counterproductive.

The FDA banned health benefit claims related to alkaline water due to insufficient evidence. Small studies suggest minor benefits for acid reflux and bone density, but these are preliminary and don't justify the hype. Most claimed benefits—anti-aging, disease prevention, improved metabolism—lack scientific backing.

Potential downsides of long-term alkaline water consumption (pH >9.8): hyperkalemia (excess potassium), mineral depletion, nutrient absorption interference, and excessive thirst.

Verdict: Save your money. Regular water hydrates just fine. If you want better water, invest in proper purification, not pH manipulation.

Myth 2: "Warm Water on Empty Stomach Cures All Diseases"

WhatsApp forwards insist warm water in the morning flushes toxins, boosts metabolism, aids digestion, prevents cancer, and possibly achieves world peace.

The reality: Warm water is...warm water. It doesn't "flush toxins"—your liver and kidneys do that regardless of water temperature. It doesn't "boost metabolism" beyond the negligible thermogenic effect of bringing water to body temperature. It doesn't prevent disease.

Drinking water (any temperature) on waking is beneficial because you're dehydrated after 7-8 hours of sleep. The temperature is personal preference, not medical necessity. Warm water may feel soothing if you have congestion or prefer it. That's it.

Myth 3: "RO Water Removes All Minerals and Is Harmful"

This myth claims RO-purified water is "dead water" devoid of essential minerals, causing deficiencies.

The reality: Yes, RO removes minerals—including calcium and magnesium. But you get 90%+ of your minerals from food, not water. A glass of milk provides more calcium than 50 liters of hard water. Your diet matters infinitely more than dissolved minerals in water.

Modern RO systems include mineralizers that add back beneficial minerals post-purification. If you're concerned, eat a balanced diet. The minerals removed by RO are negligible compared to dietary intake.

What RO *does* remove—fluoride, arsenic, nitrates, heavy metals—can literally poison you. The tradeoff is obvious and worthwhile.

Myth 4: "Stored Water Becomes Toxic After 24 Hours"

Another forward insists water stored in bottles or tanks becomes "toxic" and must be replaced daily.

The reality: Water doesn't spontaneously become toxic. Microbial growth is possible if water is contaminated and stored at warm temperatures, but properly purified and stored water lasts days. The real issue is *how* water is stored—plastic bottles exposed to sunlight can leach chemicals (BPA, phthalates) over time. Glass or food-grade stainless steel containers avoid this.

If your stored water develops an odor or taste, or looks cloudy, then yes, discard it. But 24 hours is arbitrary nonsense.

The Policy Critique: Standards That Don't Protect

India's drinking water quality standards (BIS 10500:2012) set permissible limits, but these are often inadequate:

- India's nitrate limit: 45 mg/L
- WHO recommendation: 50 mg/L (similar)
- India's fluoride limit: 1.5 mg/L
- WHO recommendation: 1.5 mg/L (same)

But here's the issue: permissible limits represent *acceptable contamination levels*, not safety. Populations drinking water within these limits still show health impacts. Lower limits would be healthier but politically and economically challenging to implement given India's water reality.

Additionally, monitoring is inadequate. Only 101 of 131 non-attainment cities have continuous air quality monitoring. Water quality monitoring is similarly sparse. Surveillance is poor, underestimating disease burden. You can't solve problems you don't measure accurately.

The Jal Jeevan Mission aims to provide tap water to all rural households, reaching 77% of 193 million households as of 2024. But experts note many pipes aren't functional, and water quality isn't always assured. Infrastructure without quality control is theater, not progress.

The Thought Experiment: If Water Were Actually Valued

Imagine if India treated water as the existential resource it is rather than a cheap, infinite commodity to be wasted and polluted at will. How would society change?

Pricing Reality

Water is absurdly underpriced in India. Urban households pay ₹5-20 per 1,000 liters of municipal water. Farmers get irrigation water essentially free. This creates no incentive for conservation.

If water were priced to reflect scarcity and treatment costs—say ₹100-200 per 1,000 liters—consumption would plummet. Wasteful practices (washing cars with hoses, overwatering lawns, excessive irrigation) would stop immediately. Industries would invest in recycling. Agriculture would shift to efficient drip irrigation from flood irrigation.

The political reality: water price increases trigger riots. So we continue subsidizing waste while aquifers deplete.

Agricultural Reform

Agriculture consumes 80-90% of India's water. Four crops—rice, wheat, sugarcane, cotton—use 700 billion cubic meters annually (60% of usable water). India uses 2-3 times more water per ton of crop than developed nations.

Rice and wheat cultivation is sustained by government minimum support prices (MSP) guaranteeing purchase at above-market rates. This incentivizes water-intensive crop production even in water-scarce regions. Punjab and Haryana grow rice—a crop requiring flooded fields—despite being semi-arid. Groundwater extraction exceeds recharge, causing wells to fail.

Reform possibilities:

- Shift MSP incentives toward water-efficient crops (millets, pulses)
- Mandate micro-irrigation (drip/sprinkler) in water-stressed regions
- Penalize excessive groundwater extraction

- Promote crop diversification based on regional water availability

India could save 200 billion cubic meters of water annually through better agricultural water management. That's enough to supply domestic needs for decades.

Political will, however, remains absent. Farmers are a powerful voting bloc. Water-intensive crops have entrenched supply chains. Reform requires courage politicians lack.

Wastewater Treatment

Currently, 70% of wastewater is untreated. Treated wastewater can be recycled for industrial use, irrigation, cooling—applications not requiring potable quality. Israel recycles 90% of wastewater; India manages barely 30%.

The government aims for 70% recycling by 2030. Achieving this requires massive investment in treatment infrastructure, piped sewage collection, and industrial wastewater regulations with actual enforcement.

Individual Actions

While systemic change requires policy, individuals can reduce water footprints:

- Dietary choices: Meat and dairy have enormous water footprints. Beef requires 15,000 liters per kg; lentils need 5,000 liters per kg. Reducing animal product consumption saves water.
- Household efficiency: Fix leaks (20% of household water is wasted through leaks), use low-flow fixtures, reuse greywater for plants.
- Conscious consumption: Every product has an embedded water footprint. Cotton t-shirts: 2,700 liters. Smartphones: 12,000 liters. Buying less means using less water indirectly.

The Home Experiment: Test Your Water

Want to understand what's in your water? Here's a simple experiment:

Week 1: Baseline Testing

Get your water tested. Don't guess. Local labs test for ₹500-2,000 and provide reports on:

- TDS (Total Dissolved Solids)
- pH
- Hardness
- Chlorine
- Nitrates
- Fluoride
- Heavy metals (if requested)
- Bacterial contamination (E. coli, coliforms)

Compare results against BIS standards. If nitrates exceed 45 mg/L, fluoride exceeds 1.5 mg/L, or arsenic is detected above 10 ppb, your water is unsafe.

Week 2: Purification Intervention

If contamination is detected, install appropriate purification:

- High TDS/chemicals/heavy metals: RO system
- Biological contamination only: UV or boiling
- Combination: Multi-stage RO+UV

Re-test water post-purification. RO should reduce TDS to 50-200 ppm and remove heavy metals/fluoride to non-detectable levels.

Observation

Track any health changes: reduction in digestive issues, skin problems, or fatigue. Often, chronic low-level contamination causes vague symptoms that disappear once exposure ends.

This experiment costs ₹1,000-3,000 but provides data. Data beats assumptions. Always.

Synthesis: Water Security as National Security

As we navigate 2025, water is transitioning from a development challenge to an existential threat. Moody's warning that water scarcity could hurt India's sovereign credit isn't hyperbole—it's a recognition that without water, economies collapse.

Agriculture employs 40% of India's workforce. Disrupting water supply disrupts food production, driving inflation, reducing incomes, and risking social unrest. Water-intensive industries—coal power, steel, textiles—face operational disruptions. Chennai's 2019 crisis saw hotels and businesses close. Scale that nationwide, and you understand the stakes.

For young Indians reading this—the engineers, doctors, entrepreneurs, policymakers-in-waiting—water will define your generation's challenges. Climate change is intensifying droughts and floods simultaneously. Population growth is increasing demand while supply stagnates or declines. Pollution is rendering existing water unusable.

Practical Actions for 2025

1. Know your water source and quality: Test it. Understand contaminants. Invest in appropriate purification.

2. Support water-positive policies: Vote for leaders prioritizing water infrastructure, wastewater treatment, groundwater recharge, and agricultural reform.

3. Reduce personal water footprint: Fix leaks, efficient appliances, dietary shifts toward plant-based foods, conscious consumption.

4. Advocate for pricing reform: Subsidized water incentivizes waste. Rational pricing enables conservation.

5. Rainwater harvesting: If you own property, install rainwater collection systems. Urban homes can recharge borewells or use harvested water for non-potable needs.

6. Spread accurate information: Counter WhatsApp myths with science. Share credible sources. Science literacy is water literacy.

7. Support technological solutions: Desalination, wastewater recycling, precision agriculture—these need investment and political backing.

The Final Word (Or: Why You Should Care About H_2O)

Water is the most ordinary and extraordinary substance on Earth. Ordinary because it's everywhere—covering 71% of the planet's surface. Extraordinary because its weird chemistry makes life possible, and its absence makes life impossible.

Understanding water—its structure, properties, contamination, purification, scarcity—isn't academic exercise. It's survival knowledge for 21st-century India. When your borewells run dry, when groundwater shows 10x safe fluoride levels, when waterborne disease hospitalizes your family—these are water problems, but they're also information problems.

The science is clear: hydrogen bonding creates properties no other molecule replicates. India's water is contaminated beyond safety in many regions. Purification technologies exist and work. Policy failures compound scarcity and contamination. Solutions—technical, agricultural, political—are known. Implementation lags catastrophically.

The gap between what we know and what we do is where the crisis lives. Bridging it requires collective action: individual choices, community pressure, political accountability, technological adoption, economic reform.

H_2O is just three atoms. But those three atoms, bent at 104.5°, polar and hydrogen-bonded, constitute the difference between thriving civilization and collapse. Treat them accordingly.

Now go test your water. Knowledge is power, but only if you use it. And for the love of science, stop forwarding WhatsApp myths about warm water curing diabetes. It doesn't. Physics doesn't work that way.

Cheers. With purified water, obviously.

CHAPTER 4: EARTH'S SOIL

The Ground Beneath Your Feet (Or: How We're Literally Destroying the Foundation of Civilization)

You're scrolling through Instagram, double-tapping aesthetic reels of rooftop gardens in Bengaluru and "urban farming" setups where millennials grow cherry tomatoes in repurposed paint buckets while explaining how they've "reconnected with nature." Meanwhile, your feed also shows farmers in Punjab burning crop stubble because disposing of it any other way is economically unviable, creating smoke plumes visible from space. Somewhere between these extremes lies an inconvenient truth that nobody wants to talk about because it's literally beneath our notice: 33% of India's soil is degraded, and we're losing the very foundation that feeds 1.4 billion people.

Here's the uncomfortable math: India has 115-120 million hectares of degraded land—that's 33% of our total geographic area affected by water erosion, wind erosion, salinity, and vegetation loss. Twenty-one major cities are expected to run out of groundwater by 2030, but before that happens, we'll have run out of healthy soil to grow food on. Meanwhile, the typical urban Indian's relationship with soil involves either complaining about mud on their shoes after monsoon or buying ₹500 "organic potting mix" for their balcony plants. The disconnect is so profound it would be funny if it weren't existentially terrifying.

But wait—it gets worse. A study analyzing 50 million soil samples collected across India between 2015-2019 found that over two-thirds were deficient in key nutrients like nitrogen, phosphorus, and potassium, and 85% contained too little organic carbon for functional soil ecosystems. In the 1970s, Indian farmers produced 15 kg of grain per kg of fertilizer used; by 2015, that ratio collapsed to 5 kg per kg. Translation: our soil is so depleted that we're pouring more and more chemical fertilizers into it for diminishing returns, like trying to revive a dead phone battery by plugging it into progressively more expensive chargers. It's not working, but we keep doing it anyway because, well, what else can we do?

The Science of Soil (Or: Why Dirt Is More Complex Than Your Netflix Recommendations Algorithm)

Let's start with the basics, because "soil" and "dirt" aren't synonymous despite how interchangeably we use them. Dirt is what you track into your house and your mother yells at you for. Soil is a living, breathing ecosystem more complex than most things you learned in engineering college.

Soil Composition: The Four-Part Harmony

Healthy soil consists of four major components in remarkably specific proportions:

- 40-45% inorganic mineral matter (sand, silt, clay)
- 5% organic matter (humus, decomposing organisms, microbial biomass)
- 25% water
- 25% air

Yes, half of healthy soil is literally nothing—pore spaces filled with water and air. This emptiness is crucial. Plant roots need oxygen to respire, and soil microbes need oxygen to decompose organic matter and cycle nutrients. Compact soil from heavy machinery or foot traffic reduces pore space, suffocating roots and killing beneficial microbes. Think of it like trying to breathe with someone sitting on your chest—technically possible, but suboptimal for long-term survival.

The Mineral Fraction: Not Just Rocks, But Rock Categories

The inorganic portion comes from weathered rocks broken down over geological timescales. Particle size determines soil texture, and this isn't arbitrary—it fundamentally affects water retention, nutrient availability, and root penetration:

- Sand particles: 0.1-2 mm diameter. Large pores, excellent drainage, poor nutrient retention. Think of sand as the Tinder of soil—everything moves through quickly, nothing sticks around.
- Silt particles: 0.002-0.1 mm diameter. Moderate drainage, moderate nutrient retention. The balanced middle child.
- Clay particles: <0.002 mm diameter. Tiny pores, poor drainage, excellent nutrient retention. Clay is clingy—holds onto water and nutrients intensely, sometimes too intensely.

Loam—the Goldilocks soil—has no dominant particle size, containing a balanced mixture of sand, silt, and humus. It drains well enough to prevent waterlogging, retains enough moisture to sustain plants between rainfalls, and holds nutrients without suffocating roots. It's the soil equivalent of perfectly cooked *khichdi*—simple ingredients, ideal proportions, nourishing results.

India's soil texture varies dramatically by region. Rajasthan's arid zones are sandy, leading to wind erosion. The Gangetic plains have alluvial silt-loam—agriculturally productive but vulnerable to water erosion. Coastal areas develop saline soils from seawater intrusion. Understanding your local soil texture isn't academic trivia—it determines what grows, how much water you need, and which management practices work.

Organic Matter: The 5% That Does 95% of the Work

Organic matter, called humus when fully decomposed, makes up only 5% of soil volume but is disproportionately important. It consists of:

- Living microorganisms (bacteria, fungi, protozoa, nematodes)
- Dead microorganisms in various decay stages
- Dead plant material (roots, leaves, stems)
- Dead animal material
- Microbial metabolic byproducts

A typical acre of healthy soil contains:

- 900 lbs of earthworms
- 2,400 lbs of fungi

- 1,500 lbs of bacteria
- 133 lbs of protozoa
- 890 lbs of arthropods and algae

That's over 5,800 lbs of living biomass per acre—roughly the weight of two adult elephants, except it's invisible, underground, and doing jobs we don't appreciate until they stop.

Organic matter improves soil in multiple ways:

1. Nutrient storage and release: Organic compounds contain nitrogen, phosphorus, sulfur, and micronutrients. As microbes decompose organic matter, they release these nutrients in plant-available forms. Without organic matter, nutrients leach away or get locked in forms plants can't use.

2. Water retention: Organic matter acts like a sponge, absorbing water and releasing it slowly. Soils high in organic matter need less frequent irrigation.

3. Soil structure: Organic compounds "glue" mineral particles into aggregates—small clumps with pore spaces between them. Good aggregate structure allows water infiltration, gas exchange, and root penetration. Poor structure (compacted, structureless soil) is hostile to plant life.

4. Carbon sequestration: More on this shortly, but organic matter is 50-60% carbon by mass. Storing carbon in soil removes CO_2 from the atmosphere, mitigating climate change.

Yet India's soils have 85% deficiency in organic carbon. Decades of intensive agriculture without replenishing organic matter have mined the soil's fertility. We've been withdrawing from the soil bank account without deposits, and now the account is overdrawn.

The Soil Microbiome: An Invisible Workforce of Trillions

This is where it gets genuinely mind-blowing. One teaspoon of healthy soil contains:

- 1 billion bacteria spanning thousands of species
- Several meters of fungal hyphae (thread-like fungal structures)

- Hundreds of protozoa
- Dozens of nematodes

The soil microbiome—the collective community of microorganisms living in soil—performs functions essential to life on Earth:

1. Nutrient cycling: Certain bacteria fix atmospheric nitrogen (N_2) into ammonia (NH_3) that plants can use. *Rhizobium* bacteria form symbiotic nodules on legume roots, converting N_2 gas into plant-available nitrogen. Without nitrogen-fixing bacteria, atmospheric nitrogen—78% of air—would be useless to plants, and you'd have no protein sources.

Other bacteria and fungi mineralize organic nitrogen, phosphorus, and sulfur, converting them from complex organic forms into simple inorganic ions (NO_3^-, PO_4^{3-}, SO_4^{2-}) that plant roots absorb.

2. Organic matter decomposition: Fungi and bacteria break down dead plant material, animal waste, and deceased organisms. Without decomposers, Earth would be buried under accumulating dead matter, and carbon would be locked forever in organic compounds rather than recycled.

3. Disease suppression: Beneficial microbes compete with pathogens for resources and physical space. Some produce antibiotics or enzymes that kill pathogens. *Bacillus subtilis* produces bacillomycin and antibacterial proteins that suppress pathogen spread. *Trichoderma* fungi actively combat pathogenic fungi and bacteria.

"Disease suppressive soils" have diverse bacterial communities that prevent pathogen proliferation through competitive exclusion and antimicrobial production.

4. Plant growth promotion: Certain soil bacteria produce plant hormones (auxins, cytokinins, gibberellins) that stimulate growth. *Pseudomonas* species secrete organic acids that improve soil structure and moisture retention.

5. Symbiotic relationships: Arbuscular mycorrhizal fungi (AMF) form mutualistic associations with 80% of plant species. Fungal hyphae extend far beyond root zones, accessing water and nutrients (especially phosphorus) that roots alone can't reach. In exchange, plants provide fungi with sugars from photosynthesis. It's a biological trade network

more sophisticated than most human markets.

Recent research affirms that soil microbial communities increase crop yields and resilience by improving soil texture and nutrient availability. Practices that enhance organic matter—like composting, cover cropping, and reduced tillage—promote soil microbial biomass and diversity. Conversely, excessive chemical fertilizers, pesticides, and herbicides reduce bacterial diversity and fungal abundance, weakening disease suppression and nutrient cycling.

India's natural farming movement recognizes this. Zero Budget Natural Farming (ZBNF), promoted in Andhra Pradesh and Karnataka, uses microbial cultures (*Jeevamrutham, Bijamrutham*) to enhance soil microbiome health. Studies show ZBNF significantly increases microbial biomass, promotes nitrogen-fixing bacteria and mycorrhizal fungi, and improves soil carbon sequestration.

India's Soil Crisis: The Numbers That Should Alarm You

Now let's confront the reality that should be triggering national emergency meetings but instead gets buried under economic growth statistics.

Soil Degradation: Losing Ground Literally

India's soil degradation statistics are catastrophic:

- 115-120 million hectares degraded (33% of total geographic area)
- Water erosion: 11.01% of India's land, the most significant contributor
- Vegetation degradation: 9.15%
- Wind erosion: 5.46%, particularly severe in Rajasthan's arid zones
- Desertification: 83.69 million hectares of dryland undergoing desertification, with cumulative increase exceeding 1 million hectares since 2003-05

States worst affected: Rajasthan (21 million hectares degraded), Maharashtra, Gujarat, Telangana, Andhra Pradesh, Karnataka, Tamil Nadu.

In Rajasthan, over 21 million hectares show severe degradation from wind erosion. In Tamil Nadu, 1.6 million hectares are affected by water erosion, salinity, and mass movements (landslides) in hilly regions. Unsustainable agricultural practices—excessive chemical fertilizers, improper irrigation, monoculture cropping—have contributed to soil hardening and reduced fertility.

Economic Impact: Losing Billions While Gaining Nothing

Soil erosion's global economic impact is projected to reach USD 625 billion by 2070 under a "middle of the road" climate scenario. The current global impact on agricultural productivity is estimated at USD 8 billion annually. Soil erosion rates are projected to increase 30-66% over 2015-2070 under various climate-economic scenarios.

India's specific economic losses from soil degradation aren't fully quantified, but agricultural productivity declines are measurable. The 15:1 grain-to-fertilizer ratio in the 1970s collapsing to 5:1 by 2015 represents massive efficiency loss. Farmers apply three times more fertilizer for the same yield, increasing costs while degrading soil further. It's an economically and ecologically unsustainable spiral.

Nutrient Depletion: The NPK Imbalance Crisis

Soil nutrients—particularly nitrogen (N), phosphorus (P), and potassium (K)—are essential for plant growth. The "ideal" NPK ratio for balanced nutrition is debated, but 4:2:1 is commonly cited for India.

Current reality: India's NPK usage ratio was 8.2:3.2:1 by 2012-13, reflecting massive nitrogen overuse relative to phosphorus and potassium. This imbalance negatively impacts crop yields and soil health.

But here's the complication: the 4:2:1 ratio isn't universally optimal. It varies by state, crop type, and soil fertility. Applying a uniform national standard is scientifically inappropriate yet politically convenient.

State-level analysis reveals:

- Six states overuse nitrogen: Andhra Pradesh, Assam, Bihar, Haryana, Jharkhand, Punjab
- Karnataka and Odisha: Near-optimal nitrogen levels

- Twelve states underuse nitrogen: Deficiencies range from 4.4% to 60%

For phosphorus, Haryana applies 45% more than recommended, while most states under-apply. For potassium, deficiencies are widespread, leading to long-term soil depletion.

Research shows NPK balance is critical: omitting any single nutrient causes yield reductions and soil depletion. NPK-treated plots maintain balanced nutrient profiles and sustainable yields, while nutrient-deficient treatments cause marked depletion and residual soil damage.

India's fertilizer subsidy policy, intended to promote balanced NPK use, inadvertently encouraged nitrogen overuse. The Nutrient-Based Subsidy (NBS) scheme launched in 2010 to correct this imbalance actually worsened it by making nitrogen relatively cheaper. Policy failures compound agricultural failures.

Organic Carbon Depletion: The Invisible Loss

Soil Organic Carbon (SOC) is a proxy for soil health. The 85% deficiency in Indian soils means most agricultural land lacks sufficient organic matter for functional ecosystems. This has cascading effects:

- Reduced water retention (more irrigation needed, higher drought vulnerability)
- Poor nutrient cycling (more fertilizer needed, lower efficiency)
- Weak soil structure (increased erosion, poor root penetration)
- Reduced microbial activity (less nutrient mineralization, weak disease suppression)
- Climate impact (less carbon sequestration, more atmospheric CO_2)

Soil Carbon Sequestration: Climate Solution Beneath Our Feet

Here's where soil transitions from agricultural concern to climate imperative. Soils globally store more carbon than the atmosphere and all vegetation combined. Maintaining and increasing soil carbon storage is a critical climate mitigation strategy.

The Carbon Cycle Connection

Plants absorb CO_2 from the atmosphere via photosynthesis, converting it into sugars and eventually into plant biomass (roots, stems, leaves). When plants die, this carbon enters soil as organic matter. Soil microbes decompose it, releasing some carbon back to the atmosphere as CO_2, while stabilizing the rest as humus.

Globally, fossil fuels release 9.5 billion metric tons (Gt) of carbon annually. Land ecosystems absorb 28% (2.66 Gt), with the vast majority stored in soils. Without this soil carbon sink, atmospheric CO_2 concentrations would be much higher, and warming more severe.

But soil carbon storage is bidirectional. Tilling (mechanically disrupting soil) exposes previously protected organic matter to oxygen, accelerating decomposition and releasing stored carbon as CO_2. It's estimated soils have lost 50-70% of original carbon stock due to agriculture.

Practices That Enhance Soil Carbon

Research shows multiple practices increase soil carbon sequestration:

1. No-till or reduced tillage: Minimizes soil disturbance, preserving organic matter and reducing CO_2 release. Conservation agriculture (CA) combining no-till with crop residue retention sequesters carbon by protecting soil organic carbon in aggregates.

2. Cover cropping: Planting legumes or grasses between cash crop seasons adds organic matter, fixes nitrogen, and prevents erosion. Cover crops improve soil health by increasing organic matter content.

3. Organic amendments: Adding compost, manure, biochar, or crop residues directly increases soil carbon. Organic farming can increase SOC by 40% compared to conventional farming after nine years. Even replacing 25% of inorganic fertilizer with organic amendments results in higher SOC, total nitrogen, and available nutrients.

4. Agroforestry: Integrating trees with crops adds carbon both above and below ground through deep root systems.

5. Crop rotation and diversification: Varying crops prevents monoculture-induced degradation and supports balanced microbial ecosystems.

6. Mulching: Covering soil with organic materials reduces evaporation, controls weeds, and adds organic matter as it decomposes.

Studies in India show natural farming systems like ZBNF significantly enhance soil carbon sequestration. Andhra Pradesh's ZBNF initiative aims to transition 6 million farms (8 million hectares) to natural farming by 2024. Practices using *Jeevamrutham* (microbial culture) and *Bijamrutham* (seed treatment) improve organic matter content, enhance soil structure, and increase microbial diversity.

Organic farming shows 46% greater very labile carbon pool than conventional methods. Natural farming increases carbon management index (CMI) by 47-33% compared to control and chemical fertilization alone. These aren't marginal gains—they're transformative improvements in soil health and climate mitigation potential.

The Skeptical View: Soil Carbon Isn't a Silver Bullet

It's important to note: soil carbon sequestration is valuable but not a standalone climate solution. Some research challenges the extent of its climate mitigation potential. Critics argue that soil carbon saturation limits exist, sequestration rates vary by soil type and climate, and management changes can reverse gains quickly. Additionally, increased SOC doesn't always correlate with increased crop yields, particularly in already fertile soils.

The takeaway: soil carbon sequestration is one tool in a comprehensive climate strategy, not a replacement for reducing fossil fuel emissions. But dismissing it would be equally foolish—it offers co-benefits (improved soil health, water retention, productivity) even if climate mitigation is slower than optimists claim.

Real-World Applications: Bringing Soil Science to Indian Farms

Theory is useless without practice. How do we translate soil science into actionable strategies for India's 146 million farmers?

Natural Farming and Organic Transitions

Multiple Indian states are promoting natural/organic farming:

Andhra Pradesh: Leading ZBNF adoption, targeting 100% natural farming statewide. Government support includes training, input subsidies, and market linkages.

Karnataka: Also promoting ZBNF with government partnerships.

Sikkim: India's first fully organic state, transitioning entirely to organic agriculture through traditional practices and local resource utilization.

Himachal Pradesh: Emphasizes natural farming adapted to mountainous terrain—terrace farming, organic mulching, indigenous manure.

These transitions show measurable improvements: enhanced soil fertility, increased microbial activity, better water retention, reduced input costs, improved farmer incomes. Natural farming, when implemented correctly with soil-specific considerations, outperforms conventional systems in long-term sustainability.

Precision Agriculture: Technology Meets Soil

Soil health monitoring is moving digital. Startups and research institutions are developing:

- Soil testing kits: Portable devices measuring NPK, pH, organic carbon, micronutrient levels
- Remote sensing: Satellite imagery tracking soil moisture, erosion, vegetation health
- AI-driven recommendations: Machine learning models analyzing soil data to provide customized fertilizer recommendations by field, not generic state-level guidelines

The Indian Council of Agricultural Research (ICAR) estimates 37% land degradation. Addressing this requires robust monitoring systems tracking soil degradation in real-time. Technology enables precision management—applying inputs only where needed, reducing waste and environmental impact.

Policy Framework: What's Missing

India has programs targeting soil health:

- Soil Health Card Scheme: Provides farmers with soil test results and fertilizer recommendations every 2-3 years

- National Mission for Sustainable Agriculture (NMSA): Promotes resource conservation, organic farming, integrated pest management
- Organic Farming Programs: Funded under Rashtriya Krishi Vikas Yojana

Yet implementation lags. Soil testing coverage is incomplete. Recommendations often use outdated generic ratios rather than location-specific data. Subsidies still favor chemical fertilizers over organic amendments. Enforcement of erosion control measures is weak.

What's needed:

- Stronger monitoring infrastructure: More soil testing labs, real-time degradation tracking
- Revised subsidy structure: Incentivize organic amendments, penalize practices causing degradation
- Farmer education: Training on sustainable practices, soil biology, long-term management
- Market support: Guaranteed procurement and premium pricing for organic/natural farming produce
- Research investment: Location-specific studies on optimal NPK ratios, carbon sequestration rates, microbiome management

Without political will and funding, programs remain aspirational rather than transformative.

Critical Analysis: Myths, Misconceptions, and WhatsApp Wisdom

Let's address the absurd beliefs circulating about soil.

Myth 1: "More Fertilizer = More Yield"

No. The law of diminishing returns applies emphatically. Beyond optimal nutrient levels, additional fertilizer doesn't increase yields—it harms soil, pollutes water, and wastes money.

India's collapsing grain-to-fertilizer ratio proves this. We're using more fertilizer for less grain because soil health has declined. Micronutrient deficiencies, organic matter depletion, and microbial community disruption limit how much plants can use added NPK.

The solution isn't more chemical fertilizer—it's restoring soil health through organic matter, microbial diversity, and balanced nutrition.

Myth 2: "Organic Farming Can't Feed India"

False. Studies show properly managed organic/natural farming produces comparable or superior yields to conventional systems, particularly over long timescales. Natural farming in Southeast India outperformed conventional and organic systems by enhancing soil quality. Sikkim's full organic transition didn't cause food shortages.

The challenge isn't biological capacity—it's transition period. Converting from chemically dependent soil to healthy organic systems takes 3-5 years of rebuilding microbial communities and organic matter. During transition, yields may temporarily drop before recovering. Farmers need financial support during this period, which is a policy problem, not a scientific limitation.

Myth 3: "Soil Degradation Is Reversible Overnight"

Unfortunately, no. Soil formation is extraordinarily slow—it takes 500-1,000 years to form 1 inch of topsoil under natural conditions. We've lost soil in decades that took millennia to form. While conservation practices can halt further degradation and begin restoration, full recovery to pre-degradation states requires decades of sustained effort.

This time asymmetry—fast degradation, slow regeneration—should terrify us into immediate action. Every year of continued degradation compounds future restoration challenges.

Myth 4: "Indian Farmers Don't Care About Soil Health"

Offensive and wrong. Farmers care deeply—their livelihoods depend on soil. The issue is economic constraints, lack of knowledge about sustainable alternatives, and policy structures that incentivize short-term thinking over long-term sustainability.

When fertilizer subsidies make chemicals artificially cheap while organic inputs remain expensive, when crop insurance rewards yield over soil health, when market prices don't differentiate organic from conventional produce—rational farmers optimize for immediate economics, not distant ecology.

Blaming farmers for systemic policy failures is intellectually lazy. The solution is changing incentive structures, providing education and financial support for transitions, and ensuring markets reward sustainable practices.

The Thought Experiment: What If We Treated Soil Like Infrastructure?

Imagine if India invested in soil health with the same intensity as highways or digital infrastructure. What would change?

Scenario 1: National Soil Health Mission

Launch a ₹10,000 crore program over 10 years focused on:

- Comprehensive soil testing: Every village, every farm, every year
- Subsidized organic amendments: Compost, biochar, microbial cultures at 75% subsidy
- Training programs: Every farmer receives training on soil biology, organic farming, erosion control
- R&D investment: Soil science research tailored to Indian conditions, not Western models

Expected outcomes: Restored organic carbon in 50 million hectares, reduced fertilizer dependency by 30%, increased water retention reducing irrigation needs by 20%, sequestered 50 million tons CO_2 annually.

Scenario 2: Regenerative Agriculture Mandate

Require all farms over 2 hectares to adopt at least two regenerative practices (no-till, cover cropping, crop rotation, organic amendments, agroforestry). Provide financial incentives for compliance, penalties for continued degradation.

Expected outcomes: Halted erosion on 80% of agricultural land, increased soil carbon by 1-2 tons per hectare per year, improved drought resilience, reduced fertilizer runoff into water bodies.

Scenario 3: Soil Carbon Markets

Create domestic carbon credits for verified soil carbon sequestration. Farmers earn tradable credits for increasing SOC, sold to industries needing to offset emissions.

Expected outcomes: Additional income stream for farmers practicing regenerative agriculture, market-driven incentive for soil health improvement, measurable carbon sequestration with rigorous monitoring.

These aren't fantasy—they're policy choices. The technology, knowledge, and resources exist. Political will doesn't.

The Home Experiment: Grow Your Own Soil Knowledge

Want to understand soil firsthand? Try this:

Week 1: Soil Texture Test

Materials: Handful of soil, glass jar, water, measuring tape

Method:

1. Fill jar 1/3 with soil
2. Add water until 2/3 full
3. Shake vigorously for 1 minute
4. Let settle for 24 hours

Observation: Particles settle by density. Bottom layer (sand), middle layer (silt), top layer (clay). Measure each layer's thickness to estimate texture percentages.

Week 2: Organic Matter Comparison

Materials: Two pots, poor soil (construction site dirt), good soil (garden compost-enriched), same plant species

Method:

1. Plant identical seedlings in both
2. Water equally
3. Observe growth over 2-3 weeks

Observation: Compost-rich soil supports faster growth, greener leaves, stronger stems. This demonstrates organic matter's role in nutrient availability and water retention.

Week 3: Microbial Activity

Materials: Soil sample, hydrogen peroxide (3%)

Method:

1. Place soil in container
2. Pour hydrogen peroxide on soil
3. Observe fizzing

Observation: Fizzing indicates microbial catalase enzyme activity—more fizzing means more active microbes. Compare different soils (garden vs. compacted path) to see microbial differences.

These simple experiments cost ₹100-200 but provide tangible understanding of soil properties and health indicators.

Synthesis: Soil as India's Future

We're at an inflection point. India's soil degradation trajectory is unsustainable—33% degraded now, potentially 50%+ by 2050 if current practices continue.

Food security depends on soil health. Water security depends on soil health (organic matter retains water). Climate stability depends on soil carbon sequestration. Economic prosperity depends on agricultural productivity, which depends on soil.

For young Indians—the generation inheriting both the problem and responsibility for solving it—understanding soil science isn't optional. Whether you're an agricultural engineer, policy maker, entrepreneur, or concerned citizen, soil health is your problem.

Practical Actions for 2025

1. Support regenerative agriculture: Buy organic/natural farming produce when possible. Market demand drives farmer transitions.

2. Compost organic waste: Convert kitchen scraps and yard waste into

compost. Reduces landfill waste while creating valuable soil amendment.

3. Advocate for policy change: Vote for leaders prioritizing soil health, support organizations working on agricultural sustainability.

4. Spread knowledge: Counter WhatsApp myths with science. Share credible sources, explain soil biology to friends/family.

5. If you farm or garden: Test your soil, add organic matter, minimize tillage, practice crop rotation, use cover crops.

6. Invest in soil: Whether financially (supporting regenerative agriculture startups) or politically (demanding government action), treat soil as critical infrastructure.

The Final Word (Or: Why You Should Give a Damn About Dirt)

Soil is the most underappreciated, undervalued, and under-protected natural resource we have. It took Earth billions of years to evolve the complex interplay of minerals, organic matter, water, air, and trillions of microorganisms that constitute functional soil ecosystems.

We've degraded 33% of it in a few decades. That's not a statistic—it's a crime scene in slow motion. Every ton of topsoil lost to erosion, every percentage point decline in organic carbon, every microbial species driven locally extinct—these aren't reversible on human timescales.

Understanding soil—its composition, biology, chemistry, degradation processes, restoration practices—is understanding the foundation of civilization. When soils collapse, societies follow. The archaeological record is littered with civilizations that degraded their soils and disappeared.

India doesn't have to repeat history. We have the science, technology, and resources to restore soil health. What's missing is collective will and individual action at scale.

The good news: soil is forgiving. Stop harming it, start nurturing it, and it will recover. Not overnight, not completely, but meaningfully. Every organic amendment added, every chemical fertilizer replaced, every microbial culture introduced, every tillage pass skipped—these accumulate into systemic recovery.

The ground beneath your feet is quite literally the ground beneath your future. Treat it accordingly.

Now go outside, pick up a handful of soil, and appreciate that you're holding a community of trillions working 24/7 to keep you alive. Then figure out how you're going to protect it.

Because if you won't, who will?

CHAPTER 5: MEDITATION

The Billion-Rupee Brain Hack (Or: Why Your WhatsApp Uncles Might Be Onto Something, But Not For The Reasons They Think)

Your Uncle Rajesh, the one who exclusively shares LinkedIn motivational quotes and WhatsApp forwards about ancient wisdom, messages your family group chat at 6:47 AM: "Meditation has CHANGED MY LIFE! 🧘✨ Wake up early, sit quietly, EMPTY YOUR MIND, and miracles happen. My productivity increased 500%! My salary TRIPLED! My wife now loves me again! Jai Bharat 🇮🇳"

Meanwhile, your anxiety-ridden engineering colleague from BITS Pilani, drowning in Jira tickets and Slack notifications, asks: "Does this actually work or is it just Instagram wellness nonsense?" You're scrolling through YouTube, seeing sponsored ads for meditation apps costing ₹999/month promising to "rewire your brain in 21 days" while actual neuroscience labs are publishing fMRI studies showing that meditation—particularly long-term practice—demonstrably alters your brain's default mode network, reduces mind-wandering activity, lowers cortisol levels, and improves emotional regulation through specific neural mechanisms.

Here's what you need to know: meditation isn't magic, but it's close. And unlike your Uncle Rajesh's claims, the science is legitimate. It's also not what most people think it is.

The Neuroscience of Sitting Still (Or: Your Brain Is A Badly Configured Traffic Intersection)

Let's talk about what happens in your brain when you're not trying to do anything. When you're staring at the ceiling during a boring meeting, or scrolling through Instagram for the 47th time in an hour, or stuck in Bangalore traffic contemplating life choices—your brain defaults to what neuroscientists call the Default Mode Network (DMN).

The Default Mode Network: Your Brain's Gossip Channel

The DMN is a network of connected brain regions that activate when you're not focused on external tasks. Its primary occupants are:

- Medial prefrontal cortex (mPFC): Processes self-referential thoughts—"What do people think of me?" "Why did I say that embarrassing thing in 2012?" "Do I make enough money?" Basically, the CEO of overthinking.
- Posterior cingulate cortex (PCC) and precuneus: Contributes to self-related memory and personal relevance judgments. Why that comment someone made last week still bothers you at 2 AM.
- Temporoparietal junction (TPJ): Involved in theory of mind—inferring what others are thinking. Also the source of "Did she mean that sarcastically?" spirals.

When your DMN is active, you're essentially engaged in *mind-wandering*—a state of consciousness marked by thoughts about yourself, your past, your future, and what others think. Sound familiar?

Here's the brutal reality: mind-wandering comprises roughly 50% of human waking life. For half your conscious existence, your brain is essentially playing gossip and reviewing embarrassing moments. And this incessant self-referential processing correlates strongly with unhappiness, anxiety, and depression.

What Happens During Meditation: The DMN Becomes Boring

When experienced meditators engage in meditation, something fascinating occurs: the DMN deactivates significantly compared to both novices and to other demanding cognitive tasks.

A landmark study by Brewer et al. (2011) examining experienced meditators during concentration, loving-kindness, and open awareness meditation found:

- Main DMN nodes (mPFC and PCC) were relatively deactivated in experienced meditators across all meditation types compared to controls
- Stronger coupling developed between the PCC and brain regions associated with self-monitoring and cognitive control (dorsal anterior cingulate, dorsolateral prefrontal cortex)
- This pattern was consistent with decreased mind-wandering, suggesting meditators' brains physically organize differently at baseline and during meditation

More recent research (2024) using dynamic functional connectivity analysis found that meditators don't completely "turn off" the DMN—instead, they shift to brain states involving enhanced sensory and embodied processing, particularly posterior regions of the brain (visual, dorsal attention networks). Essentially, experienced meditators stop staring inward at their own drama and start attending to the present moment.

Think of it like this: Your DMN is a Bangalore traffic intersection during peak hours, with cars (thoughts) endlessly circulating, honking about past mistakes and future anxieties. Meditation doesn't eliminate traffic—it establishes a traffic light system. You still have thoughts, but they're regulated, organized, and don't trap you in endless loops.

The Triple Network Model: When Your Brain's Management Systems Talk

Modern neuroscience conceptualizes brain activity through three major networks:

1. Default Mode Network (DMN): Self-referential, mind-wandering, past/future focus

2. Salience Network (SN): Attention-switching, emotional significance detection, interoception (sensing your internal body state). This is your "what matters right now?" filter.

3. Central Executive Network (CEN): Task focus, goal-directed behavior, working memory, executive function. This is your "get it

done" network.

Normally, these networks are somewhat antagonistic—when DMN is active, CEN is suppressed (hence why you can't focus when mind-wandering). What meditation does is fascinating: it increases functional connectivity between these networks, particularly between DMN and SN.

A 2022 study found that just 31 days of mindfulness training increased interconnectivity between DMN nodes and Salience Network nodes in meditation-naive subjects. This suggests meditation trains your brain to become aware of mind-wandering (SN activation) while the mind is wandering (DMN activation)—essentially creating a "mindful mode" where you notice what's happening without being entirely consumed by it.

Advanced meditators show even more sophisticated brain state dynamics. A 2025 fMRI study of advanced concentrative meditation practitioners identified distinct brain states: DMN-anticorrelated states (pure focus), hyperconnected states (heightened sensory awareness), and sparsely connected states (deep absorption). Experienced meditators can move between these states intentionally.

The Neurochemistry: Cortisol, Telomeres, and Staying Young(er)

Beyond network reorganization, meditation affects your body's chemistry. The primary mechanism is reducing stress hormone production, particularly cortisol.

An Indian study on Heartfulness meditation (a form taught by the Heartfulness Institute) found:

- Cortisol levels significantly decreased ($p < 0.001$) in meditators after 12 weeks compared to controls
- Anxiety and perceived stress decreased measurably
- Well-being and mindfulness increased
- Intriguingly, telomere length increased in meditators (though not significantly, $p > 0.05$). Telomeres are DNA caps that shorten with each cell division—longer telomeres correlate with longer lifespan. A negative correlation existed between telomere length and cortisol, suggesting chronic stress literally ages your

cells.

Another randomized controlled trial comparing Rajyoga meditation to music therapy for COVID-19 stressed healthcare workers found:

- Both practices reduced anxiety and stress significantly
- Well-being improved measurably
- Rajyoga was comparable to music therapy in reducing COVID-related psychological distress

The mechanism: Chronic stress activates your sympathetic nervous system (fight-or-flight), elevating cortisol, adrenaline, and inflammatory markers. Meditation shifts activation toward your parasympathetic nervous system (rest-and-digest), lowering these markers. Your body physically relaxes, and this relaxation effect accumulates over time with regular practice.

Real-World Applications: From Corporate Cubicles to Cricket Commentary

The Indian Startup Wellness Boom

India's corporate landscape has undergone a seismic shift regarding employee mental health. Multiple major corporations now include meditation programs:

Infosys: Launched HAIL (Health Assessment and Lifestyle Enrichment), offering holistic wellness including meditation, exercise, and mental health support

TCS (Tata Consultancy Services): Implemented TCS Cares, providing mental health awareness, counseling, and self-help resources. With 600,000+ employees globally, scaling wellness matters

Reliance: Offers Employee Assistance Programs (EAP) with 24/7 access to mental health tools and services

Happiest Minds: Dedicates 60 minutes weekly to guided mindfulness practices including breath-watching, sense walks, and specialized techniques

Zomato: Introduced "Wellness Leave"—employees can take a mental health day without medical certificates, resulting in 30% reduction in stress-related sick leaves

Flipkart: Integrated mindfulness and meditation sessions into employee engagement programs, contributing to 15% improvement in employee satisfaction

These aren't charitable initiatives—they're business calculations. Studies show:

- Meditation increases employee productivity by 120%
- Employers implementing meditation programs see 85% decrease in absenteeism
- Businesses with meditation programs for employees experienced 520% profit increases
- Companies with inadequate mental health support experience 20% higher turnover rates

Emerging startups are capitalizing on this trend. Companies like Psyche Health and Fitternity provide tailored meditation and wellness programs accessible via apps. AI-powered mindfulness apps are now entering the market, personalizing meditation recommendations based on individual stress levels and preferences.

The Competitive Exam Advantage

India's competitive exam culture (JEE, NEET, UPSC, CAT) creates tremendous psychological pressure. Students report extreme stress from academic expectations, parental pressure, and fear of failure.

Research shows mindfulness and meditation interventions significantly reduce exam-related anxiety:

- Mindfulness-based interventions reduce anxiety and depression in student populations
- Studies specifically on anxiety disorders show escitalopram (antidepressant) and mindfulness-based stress reduction are essentially equivalent in efficacy
- Two weeks of mindfulness training reduces mind-wandering in students prone to distraction

For students juggling engineering entrance exams, JEE prep, or competitive job interviews, 5-10 minutes of daily meditation costs nothing and produces measurable improvements in focus and anxiety management.

Depression and Anxiety: The Evidence Is Robust

A meta-analysis of mindfulness-based interventions for depression found:

- Significant overall effect on depressive symptoms (standard mean difference = −1.14, $p < 0.001$)
- Longer interventions (>8 weeks) showed better results (SMD = −1.44) versus shorter interventions (SMD = −0.90)
- Long-term benefits persisted at follow-up (SMD = −1.28)

For anxiety specifically, a large study (n=1,151) examining the mechanisms through which mindfulness reduces anxiety found:

- Mindfulness reduces anxiety directly and indirectly through emotional regulation mechanisms
- Worry and rumination were the most potent mediators—mindfulness helps you stop mentally time-traveling to worst-case scenarios
- Meditation practice increases mindfulness, which then reduces anxiety—it's a skill you develop, not instant relief

Important caveat: meditation isn't a substitute for professional mental health treatment. For clinical depression or anxiety disorders, meditation should complement (not replace) therapy and/or medication.

Critical Analysis: Debunking Meditation Mythology

Now let's address the absurd myths circulating about meditation, often spread by wellness influencers, WhatsApp forwards, and self-help gurus.

Myth 1: "Empty Your Mind Completely"

This is perhaps the most counterproductive meditation myth. Many people attempt meditation, have thoughts appear within 30 seconds, declare themselves "bad at meditation," and quit.

The reality: Meditation is not about achieving complete mental silence.

Thoughts are inevitable—your brain generates roughly 60,000 thoughts daily. The goal is awareness without judgment.

Meditation is observing thoughts like clouds passing through the sky, not eliminating the sky. When you notice your mind wandered (and it will), you gently redirect attention back to your breath or chosen focus. That redirection is the practice. You're training attention, not eliminating consciousness.

Myth 2: "You Must Meditate for Hours"

False. Research clearly shows even 5-10 minute sessions produce measurable benefits. Consistency matters more than duration.

Two weeks of mindfulness training (duration not specified but presumably brief sessions) reduced mind-wandering in distraction-prone participants. Thirty-one days of daily mindfulness training altered large-scale brain network connectivity.

The problem: many people conflate intensity with efficacy. You can't cram meditation—it's like physical fitness. Daily 10-minute walks outperform sporadic marathon running.

Myth 3: "You Need a Perfect, Quiet Environment"

While a quiet space enhances practice, it's not mandatory. Meditation can be practiced in noisy offices, crowded homes, public parks, Bangalore traffic jams.

The skill develops gradually—initially, quiet helps. With consistent practice, meditators maintain meditative states in distracting environments. Your brain develops noise-filtering ability.

Myth 4: "Meditation Is A Quick Fix For Stress"

Meditation provides immediate relief—even a single 10-minute session reduces stress acutely. But sustained benefits require regular practice.

Think of meditation as mental fitness: occasional exercise helps, but habit transforms your baseline physiology. With consistent practice, you develop resilience—not elimination of stress, but improved responses to it.

Myth 5: "Only Spiritual People Meditate"

Completely false. While meditation originates in spiritual traditions (Buddhism, Hinduism, Taoism), it's a secular neuroscientific tool. You can be a atheist engineer practicing mindfulness meditation—the neural mechanisms function independently of spiritual beliefs.

The Limitation: Meditation Isn't Magical

Here's where I need scientific honesty: some claims about meditation are overstated:

- Some studies show no significant effect on cognitive function in certain populations
- Meta-analyses find meditation's effects on mental health are "small to moderate," not transformative
- Positive affect and well-being show limited evidence of improvement in some studies
- Publication bias likely inflates perceived benefits—studies showing positive results get published, negative studies languish

Additionally, research quality varies. Many studies lack proper sham meditation controls or employ small sample sizes. Some findings from high-quality RCTs suggest smaller effects than popularized claims suggest.

Accurate framing: Meditation significantly improves anxiety, depression, and stress in most populations when practiced consistently, with effect sizes ranging from small to moderate. It's evidence-based, but not magical. It complements but doesn't replace professional mental health treatment.

The Thought Experiment: Your Brain's Operating System

Imagine your brain as a computer with an operating system running continuously in the background. This OS (Default Mode Network) runs maintenance processes—reviewing past experiences, planning futures, simulating social scenarios.

Normally, this OS runs 24/7, consuming battery (your mental energy) even when you're not running any applications. You're constantly processing social dynamics, worrying about acceptance, replaying conversations—all unconsciously.

Meditation is essentially rebooting this system. You're deliberately pausing the background processes and directing attention to the present moment (the active application—breathing, sensing, being).

Initially, this is difficult. Your system is accustomed to background DMN processing—it feels natural, almost compulsive. But with practice, two things happen:

1. You develop awareness of DMN activity (the Salience Network activates to notice mind-wandering)
2. You reduce identification with these thoughts—they're processes, not truth

Over time, your system becomes more efficient. Background processes still run (you can't eliminate them), but they consume less battery. Your conscious attention becomes more available for present-moment activities rather than being hijacked by self-referential loops.

This isn't metaphorical—neuroimaging shows these exact changes.

The Home Experiment: Meditation for Skeptics

Want to test this without committing to spiritual practice? Here's a protocol:

Week 1: Baseline Assessment

- Rate your stress on a 1-10 scale daily
- Track your mood (happy/anxious/neutral)
- Note your focus quality (can you concentrate for 25 minutes without phone?)
- No meditation yet—just measurement

Week 2-4: Intervention

- 10 minutes daily, focusing on breath. Inhale for 4 counts, hold for 4, exhale for 4. When your mind wanders (it will), notice it without judgment and return to breath
- Continue daily tracking

Week 5: Comparison

- Re-rate stress levels
- Assess mood changes

- Evaluate focus quality

Most people report noticeable improvements: reduced anxiety, better focus, slightly better mood. The effect is real, measurable, and reproducible.

The skeptical engineer in you will appreciate this: it's self-designed, quantified, and falsifiable.

Synthesis: Why This Matters for India's Future

India faces a mental health crisis of epic proportions. NIMHANS and industry surveys show 45% of young professionals in startups experience high stress levels, with 60% reporting burnout. Depression and anxiety are becoming the default mental states for competitive exam students, corporate professionals, and startup founders.

Traditional solutions—therapy, medication—remain inaccessible for most Indians due to cost, stigma, and limited mental health infrastructure. Meanwhile, Western wellness culture is flooding Indian social media with ₹999/month meditation apps promising unrealistic transformation.

Meditation occupies a unique middle ground: scientifically validated, free or cheap, culturally rooted (ancient Indian practice), and scalable. If India systematized meditation-based wellness in schools, colleges, and corporate environments, the mental health impact would be profound.

Practical implications for young Indians:

1. School/College: Implement mandatory mindfulness training. Even 10 minutes before exams reduces anxiety and improves performance. Cost: essentially zero if using trained faculty.

2. Startups: Corporate meditation programs show demonstrable ROI—120% productivity increase, 85% reduced absenteeism, significant retention improvements. No-brainer business case.

3. Personal mental health: For stress, anxiety, sleep issues, and focus problems, meditation is evidence-based, free, and has no side effects. Try it before pursuing pharmaceutical solutions.

4. Tech innovation: AI-powered meditation apps personalizing practice recommendations—an Indian startup opportunity in global wellness market.

The irony: India invented meditation thousands of years ago, lost connection to it during colonization and industrialization, and is now "rediscovering" it through Western neuroscience. Your ancestors weren't wasting time sitting quietly—they were optimizing their neural architecture.

The Final Word (Or: Why You Should Meditate Despite Your Instincts)

Meditation appears deceptively simple—sit still, breathe, observe thoughts. For achievement-oriented Indians trained to optimize, produce, and excel, doing nothing feels wasteful. But neuroscience reveals that "doing nothing" physically reorganizes your brain, reducing the very mind-wandering that causes anxiety and depression.

You're not wasting time—you're debugging your nervous system. You're teaching your brain to distinguish between genuine threats requiring fight-or-flight responses and self-generated anxiety loops that aren't actually dangerous.

Here's the scientific truth: You spend 50% of your waking life in mind-wandering, self-referential thought patterns that correlate with unhappiness. Your brain's Default Mode Network is essentially a gossip channel broadcasting constantly about your inadequacies, mistakes, and future catastrophes. Meditation is the off switch—not an off-OFF switch, but a volume control.

The evidence is overwhelming: consistent meditation practice reduces anxiety and depression (effect sizes: small to moderate), improves stress resilience (cortisol reduction, objective biomarkers), and doesn't hurt anyone. It's evidence-based, it's free, and—unlike your Uncle Rajesh's claims—it won't triple your salary overnight. But it will improve your mental baseline, focus quality, and emotional resilience.

Is that not worth 10 minutes daily?

Now stop reading, sit somewhere quiet(ish), and try this: breathe in for

4 counts, hold for 4, exhale for 4. When your mind wanders (it will), smile at the thought, notice how funny it is that you can't even sit still for two minutes, and gently return to breathing. Repeat for 10 minutes.

Congratulations. You've just activated your Salience Network, partially deactivated your Default Mode, and slightly reorganized your prefrontal-limbic connectivity.

Your brain is already changing.

Welcome to meditation. It's not magic, but it's the closest thing neuroscience has to offer.

CHAPTER 6: PRAYERS & MANTRA

The Sacred Sound That Neuroimaging Can't Quite Explain (But Is Trying Really Hard)

Your grandmother insists you chant the Hanuman Chalisa every morning—it's "good for the soul" and "protects you from negativity." Your friend from BITS sent you a ₹999/month Calm app subscription with a message: "Try this Transcendental Meditation, bro. Completely scientific. Your amygdala will thank you." Meanwhile, you're scrolling through LinkedIn where someone just posted: "I started praying daily 6 months ago and my business DOUBLED! The universe is listening! 🙏✨" and your BS detector is screaming.

Here's what you need to know: that grandmother, that app algorithm, and that LinkedIn guy are accidentally onto something. But also—they're mostly full of it. The science behind prayer and mantras is simultaneously more boring and more fascinating than spiritual claims suggest. No, the universe isn't personally monitoring your WhatsApp status and rewarding you for consistency. Yes, repetitive vocalization measurably reorganizes your brain in ways that reduce anxiety and stress. Yes, there's actual neuroscience happening. But also, the mechanisms are complicated, the claims are often exaggerated, and—most importantly—the effects depend entirely on how you do it, not magical thinking.

Let's separate the genuine neuroscience from the Instagram wellness fiction.

The Neuroscience of Repetitive Sound (Or: How Your Brain Gets Bored Into Relaxation)

When neuroscientists first decided to study mantra chanting using functional MRI machines, they got a genuinely unexpected result. Repetitive speech—simply repeating a single word, completely divorced from spiritual context or meditation training—caused widespread deactivation across the brain's default mode network.

The Mantra Effect: Global Inhibition

A landmark fMRI study by Berkovich-Ohana et al. (2015) examined 23 non-meditators covertly repeating a single word while lying in an MRI scanner. The results were surprising:

The repetitive speech induced widespread reduction in brain activity, particularly in the default mode network (DMN) associated with self-referential thought and mind-wandering. But here's the critical part: unlike most cognitive tasks where reduced activation in one area corresponds with increased activation elsewhere, the repetitive speech resulted in unidirectional negative activity—brain regions simply shut down without compensatory activation elsewhere.

The DMN—remember from the meditation chapter?—is your brain's gossip network, active when you're thinking about yourself, your past, your future, what others think of you. When you repetitively chant a mantra, you're essentially forcing your brain's self-referential processing systems into silence.

Importantly, this happened in non-meditators, people with zero meditation experience. The "mantra effect" doesn't require spiritual belief, meditation expertise, or understanding Sanskrit. It's a neurobiological consequence of repetitive sound.

The mechanism proposed is called "global gating"—the minimally demanding repetitive speech triggers a widespread inhibition of cortical activity. Think of it like your brain receives the message: "Oh, you're just going to repeat the same thing? Cool. I'm going to stop micromanaging everything and just... chill.".

EEG Correlates: Brain Waves During Chanting

While fMRI shows what's shutting down, EEG (electroencephalography) measures the electrical oscillations—brain waves—during mantra practice. Studies consistently show similar patterns across different chanting traditions:

Alpha wave increase (8-12 Hz, associated with relaxation and calm attention): Multiple studies show elevated alpha during and after mantra chanting. A study on Mahā Mantra (Hare Krishna) chanting found statistically significant increase in alpha power post-chanting ($p < 0.001$).

Theta wave modulation (4-8 Hz, associated with meditation and drowsiness): Extended mantra practice increases frontal theta, indicating sustained attention and focus.

Beta wave reduction (13-30 Hz, associated with active thinking and problem-solving): Decreased beta during chanting correlates with reduced cognitive demand and mental effort.

The pattern—increased alpha and theta, decreased beta—is essentially the brain's signature of relaxation. OM chanting specifically shows enhanced parasympathetic nervous system activity within 5 minutes, literally activating your body's "rest-and-digest" response.

Prayer: A Different Neural Signature

Here's where it gets interesting. Prayer—particularly religious prayer where you're addressing a deity—shows a different fMRI signature than mantra chanting. A study of Sahaja Yoga practitioners during formalized prayer versus secular speech found:

- Bilateral thalamus deactivation during prayer (but not secular speech), suggesting decreased external sensory processing—essentially "tuning out" the world
- Reduced activity in medial prefrontal cortex regions involved in social cognition
- Frontal region deactivation suggesting less "mentalizing" (inferring what others are thinking)

This differs from mantra chanting's widespread DMN shutdown. Prayer seems to specifically suppress theory-of-mind and social judgment regions while simultaneously dampening external awareness.

If mantra is "turning down the noise," prayer is "redirecting attention inward while stopping social judgment processes."

A broader literature review found prayer activates specific circuits involved in attachment and social reward, which might explain why prayer can feel emotionally resonant versus mantras' more "mechanical" relaxation effect. Prayer involves relationship—with God, the divine, or spiritual entities. Mantras involve repetition. Different pathways, similar endpoints.

The Importance of Sound Itself: Beyond Words

An important caveat: these effects aren't purely psychological. Sound itself—vibration—has physical effects on human systems:

Hemodynamic effects: Low-frequency sound (up to 250 Hz, including infrasound 1-16 Hz) stimulates endothelial cells and affects blood flow.

Neurological effects: Sound waves activate protein kinases in neurons and may stimulate specific nerve pathways, particularly relevant for sound's analgesic (pain-reducing) effects.

Musculoskeletal effects: Vibration affects bone cell behavior, potentially influencing bone density and spinal health.

When you chant OM, you're producing frequencies (roughly 136 Hz and harmonics) that literally vibrate your body. The vagus nerve—your major parasympathetic "rest" nerve—has auricular (ear) branches. Some research hypothesizes that OM's vibrations directly stimulate these vagal branches. This isn't mystical energy—it's acoustic stimulation of a specific nerve system.

Recent research suggests OM chanting might also enhance cerebrospinal fluid flow and metabolic waste removal in the brain through mechanical vibration effects. This has implications for neurodegenerative disease prevention, though current research is preliminary.

Real-World Applications: From Corporate Stress to Clinical Mental Health

Prayer and Religious Practice in India's Mental Health Crisis

India has a mental health crisis. The 2016 National Mental Health Survey reported 5.1% prevalence of common mental disorders (depression, anxiety). Among youth, this is significantly higher—particularly among competitive exam students and startup employees. Yet mental health infrastructure is abysmal: roughly 1 psychiatrist per 1,500,000 people in rural areas.

Religious and spiritual practice—including prayer and mantra chanting—serves as accessible, low-cost mental health intervention for millions. A large Indian study examining 31,464 older adults found that religiosity and religious participation moderately reduced the relationship between depression and cognitive impairment. Among older adults with depressive symptoms, those engaging in religious activities had lower risk of cognitive decline.

During COVID-19, researchers found that positive religious coping was significantly associated with lower stress. An Indian survey during the pandemic found over 50% reported increased spirituality. Prayer shifted from periodic observance to daily coping mechanism.

The mechanism: Prayer and mantra practice activate parasympathetic systems, reduce cortisol (stress hormone), enhance emotional regulation, and provide meaning-making—all evidence-based therapeutic tools. They're not replacing therapy or medication, but they're accessible interventions with demonstrated benefits.

Corporate Wellness Applications

Indian startups and tech companies are increasingly incorporating meditation and prayer-adjacent practices (breathwork, mindfulness) into employee wellness. While mantra-specific corporate programs are less common than general meditation apps, the underlying mechanisms apply: companies providing space for contemplative practice see benefits.

OM chanting studies specifically show:

- 5-minute sessions reduce blood pressure in hypertensive patients
- Improved heart rate variability (marker of cardiovascular health)

- Reduced anxiety and depression scores with regular practice
- Enhanced focus and cognitive function in students

Clinical Applications: Beyond Lifestyle Enhancement

Research is exploring mantra-based interventions for clinical conditions:

Anxiety and Depression: Meta-analyses show meditation and mantra practices have moderate effects on anxiety and depression comparable to some pharmacological interventions. They're not replacements for clinical treatment but valuable adjuncts.

ADHD: OM chanting has been proposed for attention improvement—its effects on frontal theta wave activity theoretically improve attention control.

Hypertension: Multiple studies show OM chanting reduces blood pressure through parasympathetic activation.

Cognitive Decline: In the Indian study of older adults, religious engagement provided moderate protection against cognitive impairment even among those with depression. This suggests prayer/mantra might be neuroprotective.

Sleep Disorders: OM chanting activates parasympathetic nervous system and reduces neural activity patterns associated with insomnia.

None of these are cure-alls. All require consistent practice. But they're scientifically legitimate, low-cost interventions in a country desperately short of mental health resources.

Critical Analysis: Where the Science Ends and Woo Begins

Now let's address the nonsense.

Myth 1: "Frequency Mysticism" and the ₹999 Apps

Your Instagram feed is flooded with claims about "432 Hz healing frequencies," "528 Hz miracle tones," and apps promising to "reprogram your DNA through sacred frequencies."

The reality: Low-frequency sound does have physiological effects (documented above). BUT:

- Specific frequency claims lack rigorous evidence. While 40 Hz gamma oscillations correlate with focused attention, and 10 Hz alpha correlates with relaxation, claiming "432 Hz specifically heals your chakras" has no scientific basis.
- The "62-70 Hz optimal health frequency" is pseudoscience. Cells vibrate at various frequencies depending on function. No universal health frequency exists.
- Sound therapy is real; frequency-specific healing is marketing. Sound *generally* affects physiology; specific frequencies don't have the magical targeting these apps claim.

The apps charging ₹999/month are selling repackaged relaxation (which works) wrapped in frequency pseudoscience (which doesn't).

Myth 2: "Mantras Reprogram Your DNA" / "Change Molecular Structure"

Repeating a mantra doesn't directly alter your genetic code. It's possible that chronic stress impairs gene expression through epigenetic mechanisms, and reducing stress through mantras could normalize that expression. But claiming mantras "reprogram DNA" is scientifically inaccurate.

The actual mechanism: Mantras reduce cortisol, enhance parasympathetic tone, reduce inflammatory markers—all of which *support* optimal cellular function. That's sufficient and impressive without DNA-hacking claims.

Myth 3: "Prayer/Mantras Cure Disease"

No. They're supportive therapies. Studies on prayer for cancer, serious illness, etc., show either null results or very small effects. Prayer has been shown to help people *cope* with illness, reduce psychological distress, and potentially improve compliance with medical treatment—not to cure pathology.

The conflation is dangerous. Someone stopping cancer treatment for prayer instead of chemotherapy isn't making a scientifically sound choice.

Myth 4: "Daily Prayer Infinitely Improves Mental Health"

Research actually shows a curvilinear relationship: people praying moderately experienced the best mental health outcomes, while those praying daily and those not praying at all had worse outcomes. This suggests:

1. Prayer helps coping but excessive prayer might indicate underlying anxiety
2. Daily prayer might reinforce worry (constant petitioning to address problems) rather than reducing it
3. Like any practice, dose and type matter

Prayer isn't an infinite benefit scaling with frequency.

Myth 5: "Specific Mantras Have Specific Powers"

Some claims: Hanuman Chalisa gives courage, Krishna mantras give devotion, etc. Neurologically, repetitive vocalization generally produces similar effects regardless of mantra content. A study comparing Om to other single-word repetition found equivalent DMN deactivation. The *meaning* you ascribe might matter psychologically (through expectancy effects), but neurobiologically, the repetition itself is the active ingredient.

This doesn't invalidate cultural/spiritual significance—meaning matters for psychological benefit. But the neural effects are largely content-neutral.

The Publication Bias Problem

Much mantra research comes from Indian institutions studying Indian traditions (excellent for cultural validity). However, these studies often show dramatic positive findings without adequate control conditions or blinding. Studies published in high-impact journals with rigorous methods show more modest effects.

The implication: mantra and prayer work better than nothing and comparable to some therapeutic interventions, but not as dramatically as much published literature suggests.

The Thought Experiment: Prayer as Neurotechnology

Imagine if prayer and mantra chanting were completely divorced from religious context and rebranded as "neurotechnology." Instead of "Om meditation," call it "Frequency Entrainment Protocol 136." Instead of "Prayer," call it "Directed Attention Retraining with Social Cognition Modulation."

Would it be more acceptable? More credible? The science would be identical—widespread DMN shutdown, parasympathetic activation, stress hormone reduction. But framed secularly, it might reach skeptical engineers and scientists who dismiss the spiritual framework.

This is actually happening: secular mindfulness apps, neurofeedback-framed meditation, sound bath "therapy" are all repackaging ancient practices in contemporary language. Sometimes the repackaging helps adoption. Sometimes it obscures that these practices have centuries of cultural context that's being stripped away.

The question for young Indians: Do you value the spiritual/cultural lineage (practicing Hanuman Chalisa as a Ramayan devotee does) or the neurological effect (chanting any mantra to reduce anxiety)? Both are valid. But they're different practices with different implications.

The Home Experiment: Mantra Efficacy Check

Design a personal test of whether mantras actually work for you:

Week 1: Baseline (no intervention)

- Daily anxiety rating (1-10 scale)
- Sleep quality (1-10)
- Focus/concentration during work (1-10)
- Resting heart rate (measure in morning)

Week 2-4: OM Chanting Intervention

- 10 minutes OM chanting daily (can be silent or audible, doesn't matter)
- Continue anxiety, sleep, focus, heart rate measurements

Week 5: Comparison

- Did anxiety decrease?
- Did sleep improve?

- Did focus improve?
- Did resting heart rate decrease?

Important: Expectancy effects are real. You might see improvements just from believing it works. That's not fake—that's psychology working alongside neurobiology. The question isn't whether you'll feel different (you might), but whether objective measures (heart rate, sleep patterns) change independent of belief.

Most people report modest subjective improvements and some objective changes (lower resting heart rate, better sleep). If you don't, you've gained clarity that it's not your intervention.

Synthesis: Prayer and Mantras in Modern India

For a generation of Indians facing unprecedented stress—competitive exams, startup culture, corporate burnout, pandemic anxiety, social media pressure—accessible stress-reduction tools matter. Prayer and mantra chanting are culturally embedded, free (or cheap), and evidence-supported.

What science validates: Mantra chanting reduces anxiety, lowers stress hormones, activates parasympathetic (relaxation) systems, improves sleep, and enhances focus. Prayer provides meaning, community, and emotional regulation benefits. Both are evidence-based interventions.

What science doesn't validate: Specific frequencies curing diseases, DNA reprogramming, manifesting wealth through prayer frequency, mantras being infinitely more beneficial with daily practice, prayer curing serious illness.

The practical implication: If your grandmother recommends daily Hanuman Chalisa chanting, she's accidentally giving sound mental health advice supported by neuroscience. If you hear claims about "528 Hz DNA activation," that's marketing pseudoscience on actual neurobiological effects. Your grandmother intuitively understood something neuroscience is now validating—repetitive vocalization with spiritual meaning reduces psychological stress and improves wellbeing.

The irony: Indians have been optimizing mental health through mantras for thousands of years. Western neuroscience spent the last 50 years "discovering" why it works. The wisdom was never absent—it was just explained through different frameworks (spiritual instead of neurobiological).

Practical Actions for 2025

1. If you're religious/spiritual: Your prayer practice likely provides genuine mental health benefits. Science validates what you've experienced. Continue, but be wary of overstated claims about miraculous healing.

2. If you're secular/skeptical: Mantra and prayer effects don't require belief. Even atheists benefit from OM chanting through parasympathetic activation. Try it purely as "stress-reduction technique." The neurobiology works independently of metaphysical claims.

3. If you're anxious/stressed: 10 minutes daily of any repetitive vocalization (OM, a secular phrase, even "om" silently) can reduce anxiety markers. It costs nothing and has zero side effects. Worth trying before reaching for pharmaceutical solutions.

4. Critically evaluate claims: If someone sells you ₹999/month frequency apps promising DNA reprogramming, they're exploiting real science (sound therapy works) with fake claims (specific frequencies don't "reprogram" anything). Sound-based relaxation? Evidence-supported. Frequency mysticism? Marketing.

5. Integrate with professional care: Prayer and mantras are supplements to mental health treatment, not replacements. If you have clinical depression or anxiety disorder, see a therapist/psychiatrist. Add mantras as complementary practice, not substitution.

The Final Word (Or: Why Science and Spirituality Aren't Actually Enemies Here)

For centuries, prayer and mantras were explained through spiritual frameworks—divine connection, cosmic vibration, spiritual elevation. Science explained them through neural mechanisms—DMN deactivation, parasympathetic activation, stress hormone reduction. These aren't contradictory. They're different descriptions of the same phenomenon at different levels of analysis.

Your spiritual practice activates specific neural circuits (scientific description). That activation feels meaningful and sacred (spiritual description). Both are true. Science doesn't diminish the significance of spiritual experience by explaining its mechanisms any more than understanding the chemistry of love diminishes falling in love.

For young Indians, this convergence is powerful. You can access ancient wisdom through cultural roots (family mantra tradition) or through contemporary neuroscience (meditation app with biofeedback). You can maintain spiritual meaning or strip it away. The underlying human capacity—repetitive vocalization's profound effects on your nervous system—remains accessible regardless.

The mantra effect is real. Prayer's benefits are real. Not because they violate physics or reprogramme DNA—because they optimize your nervous system through mechanisms evolution has gifted us.

Now, before you close this chapter, try this: Close your eyes and chant "Om" (or silently repeat "peace" or "calm"—the content doesn't matter) for 10 minutes. Feel your nervous system shift. Notice your anxiety decrease, your heartrate slow, your mind quiet.

That's not magic. That's neuroscience. Which is, arguably, more beautiful than magic because it's real, reproducible, and available to anyone willing to try it.

ॐ

CHAPTER 7: SELF-DISCPLINE (TAPAS)

The Most Boring Superpower (Or: Why Your 5 AM Gym Resolution Will Fail According To Neuroscience)

It's January 2nd, and your Instagram feed explodes with the annual "New Year, New Me" montage. Your cousin posts a selfie at a Bangalore gym with the caption: "DAY 1 OF MY TRANSFORMATION! 💪🔥 TAPAS ACTIVATED! #selfdiscipline #grind #gymlove #nofap #noporn #nosugar #nojoy". Meanwhile, you're 36 hours into your own resolution and already stress-eating maggi at midnight because your boss yelled at you during a meeting.

By January 15th, you'll have quit. So will 80% of people who made resolutions. Your cousin will post their victory photos once per week, then silently stop posting. The comment sections will be flooded with "KING" and "GOALS" from people who also failed. And everyone will blame willpower—"I don't have the discipline," "I have no self-control," "I'm just lazy."

Here's what neuroscience says: You're not lazy. Your brain is terrifyingly rational, and willpower is more complicated than social media gurus suggest. Self-discipline, *tapas* in Sanskrit—literally "heat" or "austerity"—isn't an infinite resource you can access with enough motivation. It's a negotiation between competing neural systems, constrained by glucose, contingent on context, and utterly dependent on how you frame your goals. You didn't fail because you lack discipline. You failed because nobody taught you how your brain actually works.

Let's fix that.

The Neuroscience of Self-Control (Or: Why Your Prefrontal Cortex Is A Tired Referee)

Imagine your brain as a football match between two teams: the rational, goal-oriented Prefrontal Cortex FC playing against the emotionally driven, reward-seeking Limbic System United. Self-discipline is what happens when the Prefrontal Cortex successfully constrains Limbic System's chaotic impulses. Sounds simple. It's not.

The Brain's Executive Committee: Prefrontal Cortex, Anterior Cingulate, Orbitofrontal Cortex

Your brain has dedicated regions managing self-control. The big three are:

1. Prefrontal Cortex (PFC): Located behind your forehead, this is the CEO of self-regulation. It handles decision-making, planning, and critically—inhibiting impulses. When you override the urge to check your phone during an exam, your PFC is active, literally suppressing the limbic system's "Do it now!" signal.

2. Anterior Cingulate Cortex (ACC): This region monitors conflicts between goals and competing impulses. When you're torn between studying and Netflix, your ACC is screaming, "ALERT! GOAL CONFLICT! Make a decision!" It's your internal conflict detector.

3. Orbitofrontal Cortex (OFC): Processes reward value and helps assign worth to different outcomes. When you evaluate "immediate Netflix pleasure vs. long-term exam success," your OFC is doing the math.

These three regions form the self-control network. Crucially, structural brain imaging shows that people with larger cortical volume in the right cingulate cortex demonstrate greater self-control ability. Your ability to resist temptation literally correlates with your brain's physical architecture.

But here's the catch: these are all metabolically expensive operations. Decision-making, impulse inhibition, and conflict monitoring consume enormous amounts of glucose and other neural resources.

The Ego Depletion Debate: Is Willpower Finite or Just Motivationally Fragile?

For decades, psychologists believed in the "ego depletion" model: willpower is a limited resource that depletes with use, like a phone battery. You make decisions all day, exert self-control repeatedly, and by evening, your capacity is exhausted. Hence why you binge-eat at night or doom-scroll instead of studying.

The theory was elegant. It was also wrong. Sort of.

In 2024, Baumeister et al.—the researchers who originally proposed ego depletion—issued an updated statement: the theory is more complex than originally thought. Recent failures to replicate strict depletion effects suggest the picture is nuanced.

A meta-analysis examining the interaction between motivation and depletion found something fascinating: When you're depleted, you don't *lose* willpower. You shift motivation. The compensatory effort hypothesis suggests that depleted individuals can *still* mobilize self-control if incentives are sufficient—but it requires more neural effort.

In a study tracking systolic blood pressure reactivity (a marker of mental effort), depleted participants showed the same performance as non-depleted ones when given incentives, *but with elevated brain activation in prefrontal regions.* They were working harder to achieve the same result.

Think of it like Mumbai traffic during monsoon. You're not *unable* to drive to work when the roads are flooded. You're just expending enormous effort. Most people will say "forget it" and work from home. But if your boss says "Get to the office or you're fired," suddenly you're navigating those flooded roads with maximum concentration. You didn't gain new driving ability. You shifted motivation.

The critical insight: Ego depletion isn't about lost capacity; it's about shifting motivation and conservation of resources. Your brain asks: "Is this goal worth the metabolic cost?" If the answer is no, you procrastinate.

Dopamine and Habit Formation: The Reward Prediction Error

Here's where self-discipline gets genuinely interesting, and where most people's understanding completely breaks down. Willpower isn't primarily about forcing yourself to do hard things. It's about making things feel rewarding so your brain *wants* to do them.

The mechanism is dopamine and reward prediction error (RPE). Dopamine isn't released when you *achieve* a goal. It's released when you *expect* a reward that differs from what you predicted.

Here's how it works in practice:

Scenario 1: The Unpracticed Goal
You decide to exercise. You expect it to suck (negative prediction). You do it and... it sucks. Your dopamine response is flat. Your brain records: "This matches my prediction. Neutral outcome.".

Scenario 2: The Practiced Goal With Positive Feedback
You exercise consistently. You start noticing you feel better, sleep better, look better. You complete your workout and feel accomplished. This is *better than expected.* Dopamine surges. Your brain records: "This exceeds expectations. Reinforce this behavior.".

Scenario 3: The Failed Goal
You commit to exercising. You skip the gym. You *expected* to go (positive prediction), but you didn't (negative outcome). Dopamine *crashes below baseline.* Your brain records: "This is worse than expected. I feel terrible about myself.".

The most powerful dopamine signal isn't expected rewards. It's *unexpected* rewards. If you exercise expecting it to be miserable, then discover you actually enjoyed it, that pleasant surprise generates an enormous dopamine spike. Your brain becomes motivated to repeat the behavior.

More recent research distinguishes between two dopamine systems:

1. Reward prediction error dopamine: Signals the difference between expected and actual rewards. Crucial for goal-directed behavior.
2. Movement-related dopamine: Fires during/before action

independent of reward, supporting habit formation even when rewards disappear. This explains why you keep doing things that used to be rewarding but aren't anymore—habits persist through movement dopamine signals.

The practical implication: To build self-discipline, you're not forcing yourself through will. You're organizing your environment and expectations so that disciplined behavior becomes surprisingly rewarding.

Mental Fatigue and the Frontal Cortex Sleep Response

Finally, here's where it gets alarming. A 2024 study published in *PNAS* found that prolonged mental fatigue causes the frontal cortex to exhibit EEG patterns similar to sleep, even in awake individuals. People experiencing mental exhaustion showed increased slow-wave activity (typically seen during sleep) in decision-making brain regions.

Consequence: heightened aggression, reduced empathy, and decreased cooperative behavior. Mental fatigue doesn't just make you procrastinate. It makes you *hostile.* Your brain's executive control systems literally shut down when overextended.

This partially explains why you get snappish with people when stressed (mental fatigue reducing empathy), why you make terrible decisions after long meetings (prefrontal decision-making regions in "sleep mode"), and why discipline seems impossible after exhausting days.

Real-World Applications: From JEE Aspirants to Startup Culture

The JEE/NEET Self-Discipline Requirement

India's most intense self-discipline test isn't spiritual practice. It's preparing for JEE (Joint Entrance Examination). Millions of students attempt India's most competitive engineering exam. Success requires disciplined daily work for 1-2 years with minimal immediate reward.

Research on JEE preparation identifies self-discipline as the single most critical factor, ahead of pure intelligence or access to resources. Students with strong self-discipline show:

- Improved time management: Allocating study time effectively

rather than cramming
- Sustained focus: Concentrating for extended periods without distraction
- Habit development: Establishing consistent study schedules
- Stress reduction: Adhering to routines reduces anxiety
- Persistence: Maintaining motivation through difficult periods

The research is clear but the success rate is abysmal—only ~1.2% of applicants secure JEE Main seats. Self-discipline alone isn't sufficient, but its absence is catastrophic.

Habit Formation in Digital Contexts

Indian EdTech startups are discovering what behavioral neuroscience predicted: habit formation through gamified digital interventions is dramatically more effective than passive learning.

A Stanford/Indian study examined a 100-day reading contest on an educational app for Indian children. Students who participated in the contest-based intervention showed 75% higher engagement 12 weeks after the contest ended, when external incentives disappeared. Additionally, the treatment group showed 6% increased retention in learning outcomes.

Why? Because the contest created reward prediction errors. Students expected to compete for books. They exceeded their own performance expectations. Dopamine surged. Habit consolidated.

Bangalore-based research on EdTech engagement found that gamified platforms with badges, point systems, and leaderboards increased learning participation by 45% compared to non-gamified versions. Students using apps like Forest, Habitica, or Pomodoro tools reported better time management but abandoned them without streak mechanics and peer comparison.

The pattern: Discipline, especially among young Indians, isn't intrinsic. It's environmentally scaffolded through immediate feedback, gamification, and social comparison.

Corporate Productivity and Procrastination Culture

Indian startup culture has a procrastination crisis. Early-career professionals lose approximately 30% of their time to unstructured workflows, overwhelm, and unclear prioritization. The irony: these same professionals use AI tools and productivity apps to... procrastinate more efficiently.

A common phenomenon: "productive procrastination," where you're busy but not on actual priority work—attending unnecessary meetings, organizing files, restructuring your task management system, anything except the hard work. Your brain's reward system activates from being "busy," while avoiding the discomfort of actual difficult work.

Additionally, Indian business culture's hierarchical structure contributes. Employees hesitate to make autonomous decisions, delaying projects awaiting approvals. Bureaucratic processes create systemic procrastination. This isn't personal lack of discipline—it's organizational design forcing delays.

Critical Analysis: Where Western Research Fails Indian Contexts

Myth 1: "Self-Discipline Is A Personality Trait"

Much Western psychology treats willpower as intrinsic—you either have it or don't. This is neuroscientifically wrong and culturally inappropriate for India.

Reality: Self-control capacity is influenced by context, motivation, brain structure (trainable), and environmental scaffolding. The same person can display high discipline in one domain (flawless exam prep) and zero discipline in another (staying off social media).

For Indian youth, this means: your "laziness" might not be personality. It might be misaligned motivation, environmental demotivation, or unclear expected rewards.

Myth 2: "More Discipline Solves Everything"

The "grind culture" myth: if you just work harder, sacrifice more, become more disciplined, you'll succeed. This ignores the neurobiology entirely.

Reality: Excessive reliance on self-control depletes metabolic resources, elevates stress hormones, impairs decision-making, and paradoxically reduces long-term discipline. The 5 AM gym person who forces themselves through relentless discipline often burns out by February.

Sustainable discipline requires *design*, not just effort. Structuring your environment so the right choice is the easy choice. Building habits so they're automatic, not reliant on willpower.

Myth 3: "Willpower Is Infinite If You Just Believe"

Motivational Instagram posts suggesting willpower never depletes misunderstand neuroscience. Mental fatigue is real. Prefrontal cortex resources are limited. Sleep deprivation, stress, and continuous decision-making exhaust executive function.

The solution isn't "believe harder." It's sleep better, reduce other decision demands, create environmental constraints that require less willpower.

How Western Research Doesn't Apply to Indian Conditions

Much self-discipline research uses Western university students in controlled environments with clear personal agency. India presents different constraints:

1. Systemic delays: Bureaucratic structures create forced procrastination. No amount of personal discipline overcomes procedural delays.
2. Hierarchy and deference: Cultural emphasis on respecting authority delays decision-making. Individual discipline can't overcome organizational structure.
3. Resource constraints: Limited access to quiet study spaces, unreliable electricity, internet connectivity make self-discipline more effortful than in developed nations.
4. Collectivist decision-making: Indian culture emphasizes group consensus. Individual discipline doesn't matter if you need approval from multiple stakeholders.

Western "just try harder" philosophy ignores these systemic realities.

The Thought Experiment: Designing Your Own Self-Control System

Instead of asking "How do I get more discipline?" ask "How do I design an environment where the difficult choice is the easiest choice?"

Example 1: Exam Preparation
Wrong approach: "I'll wake up at 5 AM every day and study with sheer willpower."
Right approach:

- Find a quiet study partner who also needs accountability
- Move your phone to another room (environmental design)
- Study at a library where your presence reminds you others are also studying (social pressure)
- Track hours visibly on a wall chart (reward prediction error—you see progress)
- Join a telegram group where people share solutions to daily problems (community motivation)

You're not relying on discipline. You're offloading it to systems.

Example 2: Exercise
Wrong approach: "I'll go to the gym 5 times weekly through willpower."
Right approach:

- Sign up for a group fitness class (social commitment)
- Book with a friend (accountability)
- Track your attendance publicly (reputation risk)
- Notice immediate post-workout energy boost (reward prediction)
- See physique improvements after 6 weeks (delayed but powerful positive surprise)

Again, you're creating dopamine loops and social accountability, not forcing willpower.

A Simple Five-Week Experiment

Week 1: Baseline - Pick one habit you want (exercise, study, no phone after 10 PM). Track how many days you successfully stick to it. Notice how it feels.

Weeks 2-3: Environmental Design - Restructure your environment to make the habit easier. Move your phone. Join a group. Create a visible tracker. Recruit accountability.

Weeks 4-5: Observe - Track your adherence. Most people show 40-60% improvement just from environmental change, without increased willpower.

The point: discipline isn't about forcing yourself. It's about system design.

Synthesis: Self-Discipline for India's Future

Self-discipline is traditionally framed as a moral good—virtuous effort, enduring hardship, transcending immediate comfort. *Tapas* in Sanskrit literally means the heat generated by austerity and effort.

But neuroscience suggests a different framing: Self-discipline is *rational resource management*. It's directing limited prefrontal cortex capacity toward long-term goals instead of immediate impulses.

For India in 2025, this has enormous implications:

For education: Schools teaching self-discipline as willpower alone are failing students. Effective education teaches environmental design, habit formation, and dopamine mechanics.

For startups: Indian startup culture's "grind" mythology glorifies unsustainable effort. Research shows sustainable high performance comes from systems design, not sacrifice.

For personal development: The self-help industry sells "increase your willpower" seminars. Neuroscience says: design your environment better. You don't need more discipline. You need better systems.

Practical Actions for 2025

1. Stop blaming yourself for lack of discipline. Your brain is functioning normally. Redesign your environment.

2. Understand your dopamine loops. What makes goals *feel* rewarding? Build anticipation, immediate feedback, and visible progress.

3. Create environmental constraints. Phone in another room. Study group on speed dial. Commitment devices with friends.

4. Respect mental fatigue. After exhausting days, don't expect self-discipline. Sleep, rest, reduce decision demands.

5. Measure environmental factors before blaming willpower. Hierarchy preventing you from acting autonomously? Systemic delays? These aren't personal failures.

6. For JEE/NEET/competitive exams: Use gamified platforms with streak tracking, social comparison, and immediate feedback. Don't rely on pure willpower.

The Final Word (Or: Why Discipline Isn't About Suffering)

The traditional view of *tapas*—ascetic austerity, suffering for spiritual gain—is neuroscientifically backward. You don't need more suffering. You need better design.

Your prefrontal cortex can't force behavior through willpower alone. It can architect environments that make desired behavior automatic. It can create dopamine loops that make discipline feel rewarding.

Self-discipline is often portrayed as heroic self-denial—the monk meditating in a cave, the JEE aspirant studying 14 hours daily, the startup founder sleeping at the office. Real sustainability comes from the opposite: making your environment so aligned with your values that you don't *need* willpower to stay on course.

The irony of tapas: the heat generated by austerity and effort isn't about suffering more. It's about designing your system so intelligently that discipline becomes effortless.

Waking up at 5 AM for the gym through sheer willpower? That's unsustainable.

Waking up at 5 AM because your gym buddy is picking you up, you've already paid for the class, and you track your attendance publicly? That's architecture. That's sustainable. That's real self-discipline.

Now go design your system. Your prefrontal cortex will thank you—it's exhausted from trying to run on willpower alone.

Tapas isn't about burning yourself out. It's about burning through the clutter and designing clarity.

Now excuse me, I'm going back to my distraction-proof study environment. See how easy discipline becomes when you don't rely on willpower?

CHAPTER 8: PLANTS AND HERBS (AYURVEDA)

The Ancient Pharmacy Your Grandmother Was Right About (But The Instagram Wellness People Are Mostly Wrong)

Your grandmother swears by her morning turmeric milk—*Haldi Doodh*—which she's been forcing you to drink since childhood while claiming it "heals everything" and "keeps your immunity strong." You dismissed it as placebo until you noticed she rarely gets sick and her arthritis is less severe than your grandfather's. Meanwhile, your Instagram feed is flooded with ₹2,999/month Ayurveda supplement subscriptions promising to "alkalize your body," "cleanse your dosha," and "restore your chakra balance," with testimonials from wellness influencers who also sell cryptocurrency and crypto also seems legitimate.

Here's the uncomfortable truth: Your grandmother's turmeric milk has legitimate biochemistry behind it. Curcumin, turmeric's active compound, has measurable anti-inflammatory and antioxidant properties supported by rigorous research. The Instagram supplement subscriptions are mostly expensive placebos riding on a 5,000-year-old tradition's credibility while ignoring actual evidence. And Ayurveda as a system, while containing valuable insights, has almost no rigorous clinical trial evidence compared to modern medicine—not because it doesn't work, but because historically, nobody spent money testing it rigorously.

Let's separate the grandmother wisdom from the influencer fiction, and understand what science actually says about plants, herbs, and Ayurveda in 2025.

The Phytochemistry of Traditional Medicine (Or: Why Your Body Is Basically A Chemical Factory Designed By Millions of Years of Evolution)

When modern chemistry examines Ayurvedic herbs, it finds something remarkable: plants produce extraordinarily complex molecular compounds that directly interact with human biochemistry. This isn't mystical—it's elegant chemistry.

Bioactive Compounds: Nature's Pharmacy Shelf

Ayurvedic plants don't have one magic ingredient. They have dozens, sometimes hundreds of bioactive compounds producing synergistic effects. Here's what we're actually talking about when we cite "active ingredients":

Alkaloids: Nitrogen-containing compounds with diverse pharmacological effects. Examples include:

- Berberine (from Daruharidra/Berberis aristata): Antibacterial, anti-inflammatory, improves insulin sensitivity
- Withanolides (from Ashwagandha/Withania somnifera): Stress adaptation, anti-inflammatory, potential anticancer effects
- Piperine (from Pippali/Piper longum): Enhances bioavailability of other compounds—why black pepper is added to turmeric milk

Phenolic Compounds and Flavonoids: Antioxidants that neutralize free radicals. Examples:

- Quercetin (from various plants including onions, neem): Anti-inflammatory, antihistamine, supports cardiovascular health
- Eugenol (from Lavanga/cloves, Tulsi/holy basil): Antimicrobial, analgesic, anti-inflammatory
- Curcumin (from Haridra/Turmeric): The star—potent antioxidant and anti-inflammatory, inhibits inflammatory pathways

Saponins and Glycosides: Compounds with soap-like properties and sugar-attached components with various biological effects:

- Withanosides (from ashwagandha): Adaptogenic effects, stress hormone modulation
- Asiaticoside (from Brahmi/Centella asiatica): Supports cognitive function, wound healing

Essential Oils and Terpenes: Volatile compounds contributing antibacterial and anti-inflammatory effects:

- Linalool (from Tulsi): Anxiolytic, antimicrobial
- Caryophyllene (from cloves, Tulsi): Anti-inflammatory, neuroprotective

The critical insight: these aren't magical energies or doshas realigning. They're specific molecules that bind to specific receptor sites on your cells, triggering biochemical cascades. When curcumin reduces inflammation, it's literally inhibiting COX-2 and other inflammatory pathways—the same targets anti-inflammatory drugs target. It's chemistry, not mysticism.

The Bioavailability Problem: Why Your Body Actually Uses Them (Or Doesn't)

Here's where Ayurveda's traditional combinations demonstrate actual sophistication that modern supplement companies ignore: bioavailability matters more than raw compound amounts.

Curcumin is poorly absorbed on its own—only 1-3% bioavailability. Your liver rapidly metabolizes it, and poor intestinal absorption means most is excreted. But traditional turmeric preparations always include black pepper (piperine) and fat. Why?

Piperine inhibits hepatic metabolism of curcumin AND increases intestinal absorption by up to 2,000%. Suddenly, that bioavailability jumps from 1% to 20%. Your grandmother's intuitive addition of black pepper isn't folk wisdom—it's pharmacokinetics. Fat-soluble environments increase absorption further.

This synergistic effect—where multiple compounds work together to enhance efficacy—appears throughout Ayurvedic combinations. Modern supplement companies often isolate single compounds, ignoring these interactions. The result: you're paying ₹2,999/month for suboptimally bioavailable curcumin extract.

Dose and Concentration: Why Your Grandmother's Recipe Works Better Than Instagram

An important distinction: botanical preparations don't follow pharmaceutical concentration standards. A traditional turmeric milk contains approximately 150-600 mg of curcumin per cup depending on turmeric concentration. A clinical trial dosing curcumin for inflammation typically uses 500-2,000 mg daily of standardized extract.

So traditional turmeric milk is actually... sub-therapeutic by pharmaceutical standards. Yet it works for your grandmother. Why?

Multiple reasons:

1. Chronic low-dose exposure: Daily consumption creates cumulative effects not achieved with single doses
2. Synergistic combinations: Multiple compounds work better together than isolated single compounds
3. Lifestyle integration: Turmeric milk is accompanied by other factors—sleep, family connection, cultural belief system—that activate placebo effects and stress reduction
4. Baseline inflammation levels: Chronic low inflammation (arthritis, general aging) responds better to cumulative dietary compounds than acute inflammatory conditions

The harsh reality: Instagram supplements at ₹2,999/month often contain highly concentrated, standardized extracts that are potentially more effective *on paper* for acute conditions, but lack the synergistic community, consistency, and traditional dietary integration that makes grandmother's recipe sustainable.

Real-World Applications: From Kitchen Spice to Clinical Medicine

The Evidence Landscape: What We Actually Know

Here's the problem: Ayurveda has one (1) systematic review in the Cochrane Library compared to 5 for homeopathy and 14 for Traditional Chinese Medicine. Out of 7,864 Cochrane systematic reviews, Ayurveda comprises 0.01%. This isn't because Ayurveda doesn't work. It's because nobody spent billions researching it with pharmaceutical company funding until recently.

What evidence *does* exist:

Ashwagandha (Withania somnifera): The most researched Ayurvedic herb, with measurable effects on:

- Stress and anxiety: Multiple studies show ashwagandha reduces cortisol (stress hormone) by 20-30%
- Sleep quality: Systematic review found small but significant improvement over placebo
- Cognitive function: Enhanced memory and processing speed in clinical studies, though larger trials needed
- Rheumatoid arthritis: Anti-inflammatory effects comparable to hydrocortisone in animal models; human trials ongoing
- Diabetes management: Improves insulin sensitivity in preclinical studies; human data limited

Turmeric/Curcumin (Curcuma longa): The anti-inflammatory workhorse:

- Ulcerative colitis: Two studies showed positive outcomes in disease management
- Joint pain and arthritis: Reduces inflammatory markers and pain in osteoarthritis and rheumatoid arthritis
- General inflammation: Inhibits multiple inflammatory pathways (COX-2, TNF-alpha, NF-kappa-B)

Brahmi (Bacopa monnieri): Cognitive and neuroprotection:

- Memory enhancement: Traditional use supported by studies showing improved recall and processing speed
- Anxiety reduction: Modulates neurotransmitter systems involved in anxiety regulation
- Neuroprotection: Compounds show protective effects against neurodegeneration in preclinical models

Tulsi (Ocimum sanctum): The immune herb:

- Stress adaptation: Adaptogenic effects through multiple pathways
- Immune modulation: Enhances antibody production and cellular immunity

- Anti-inflammatory: Reduces inflammatory markers in clinical studies

The honest assessment: these herbs have demonstrable effects supported by biochemistry and clinical studies, but the evidence quality is inconsistent, trial sizes are often small, and rigorous randomized controlled trials are rare.

The Indian Ayurveda Industry: Growing But Problematic

India's Ayurveda market is worth ₹10 billion USD (~₹83,000 crore) with a 16% Compound Annual Growth Rate—much faster than conventional pharma. But quality control is catastrophic:

The Heavy Metals Problem: Some Ayurvedic preparations contain dangerous levels of lead, mercury, and arsenic, particularly if prepared traditionally with metal-based medicines (rasas). The FDA has warned consumers about arsenic poisoning from Ayurvedic preparations. This isn't the herbs—it's manufacturing and traditional metal inclusion lacking modern safety standards.

The Efficacy Gap: A 2024 comprehensive review found that about 76% of patients reported complete or partial relief from Ayurvedic treatment for chronic diseases. But this is self-reported patient data from 35,000+ Indians, not randomized controlled trials. Selection bias is enormous—people already believing in Ayurveda reported satisfaction.

The Standardization Issue: Ayurvedic preparations vary wildly in phytochemical content depending on plant source, season, soil conditions, and processing methods. Your grandmother's turmeric milk from her village is biochemically different from turmeric from Andhra Pradesh, from turmeric from Peru. No standardization means no consistent dosing.

Startup Applications and Modern Integration

Indian health tech startups are beginning to bridge this gap:

- AI-driven personalization: Apps analyzing blood biomarkers to recommend Ayurvedic herbs with scientific backing
- Standardized extraction: Modern pharmaceutical techniques

ensuring consistent compound concentration while respecting traditional combinations
- Clinical validation: Startups funding rigorous trials comparing Ayurvedic preparations to conventional treatments for specific conditions

The emerging model: Ayurveda as evidence-based medicine, not tradition-based medicine. If turmeric reduces ulcerative colitis symptoms, study *why*. If ashwagandha reduces cortisol, quantify the effect size. If Brahmi enhances memory, determine the mechanism.

Critical Analysis: Separating Wisdom From Woo

Myth 1: "Ayurveda Is A Complete Medical System That Can Replace Allopathy"

Partially true. Ayurveda excels at chronic disease management, prevention, lifestyle integration, and stress-related conditions. It fails catastrophically at acute emergencies, surgical conditions, and bacterial infections requiring antibiotics.

A kidney stone doesn't care about your dosha balance. Appendicitis requires surgery, not herbal tea. Sepsis needs antibiotics. Acute myocardial infarction needs interventional cardiology. Using Ayurveda instead of evidence-based medicine for these conditions kills people.

The honest position: Ayurveda is valuable as complementary medicine and excellent for prevention. It should integrate with, not replace, conventional medicine for serious conditions.

Myth 2: "Ayurvedic Herbs Are Risk-Free Because They're Natural."

Completely false. Natural doesn't mean safe:

- Some Ayurvedic preparations contain dangerous metal concentrations (arsenic, mercury, lead)
- Herb-drug interactions are under-researched; many are potentially harmful
- Some individuals experience toxicity from Ayurvedic compounds
- Herbal preparations vary wildly in concentration, so dosing is

inconsistent

Your grandmother's turmeric milk is safe. A randomly purchased Ayurvedic supplement from a Delhi market? Significantly riskier.

Myth 3: "Dosha Imbalance Causes Disease; Rebalancing Cures It"

The pitta, vata, kapha framework is a sophisticated classification system for individual constitution and physiology. It's analogous to modern phenotyping. But the claim that "balancing your dosha" cures disease lacks any biochemical mechanism or convincing clinical evidence.

What *might* be happening: Different individuals respond differently to different herbs based on constitutional factors. A pitta constitution person might respond better to cooling herbs. A vata person to warming herbs. But this is individual variation in pharmacogenetics, not mystical dosha balancing.

The scientific reframing: Ayurveda's constitutional framework might be useful for personalizing herb selection, but the mechanism is pharmacogenomics, not energetic rebalancing.

Myth 4: "Chakra Cleansing Herbal Supplements Detoxify Your Body"

Your body has a liver, kidneys, lymphatic system, and gut microbiota designed to eliminate toxins. A supplement "detoxifying your chakra" is word salad, combining spiritual vocabulary with pseudo-scientific chemistry.

If you want liver support, use milk thistle (silymarin has hepatoprotective properties). If you want kidney support, stay hydrated and avoid nephrotoxic compounds. If you want gut health, eat fiber and fermented foods. Don't rebrand these as "chakra cleansing".

Myth 5: "Ayurvedic Standards Are Equivalent To Pharmaceutical Standards."

No. Ayurvedic preparations often lack:

- Standardized extraction procedures: Different manufacturers produce wildly different concentrations

- Quality control testing: Heavy metal testing, microbial contamination, consistency checks are inconsistent
- Clinical trial evidence: Most preparations haven't undergone rigorous human trials
- Pharmacokinetic data: Bioavailability, metabolism, excretion often unmeasured

Pharmaceutical medications are boring because they're heavily regulated. Ayurvedic preparations are exciting because they're not. But boring and safe usually beats exciting and uncertain.

The Western Research Limitation: India-Specific Factors

Much Ayurvedic research comes from India, examining Indian populations. But generalizing globally is risky:

1. Soil and climate variation: Phytochemical composition varies by geography. Indian turmeric has different compound profiles than Peruvian turmeric
2. Population genetics: Pharmacogenetic responses to herbs vary by ancestry. Effects in Indian populations may not replicate globally
3. Publication bias: Positive studies get published; negative studies languish. Indian journals may preferentially publish positive Ayurvedic findings
4. Confounding variables: Patient satisfaction in Ayurvedic studies reflects placebo effects, lifestyle changes, family support—not herb efficacy alone.

The Thought Experiment: Designing Your Own Evidence-Based Herbal Practice.

Instead of asking "Is Ayurveda legitimate?" ask "Which specific herb for which specific condition has evidence supporting it, and where should I source it safely?"

For inflammation and joint pain:

- Evidence: Curcumin (from turmeric) has moderate evidence. Ashwagandha has promising evidence
- Mechanism: COX-2 inhibition, TNF-alpha reduction, known anti-inflammatory pathways

- Dose: 500-2,000 mg curcumin daily with piperine (black pepper) for absorption
- Source: Standardized extracts from reputable manufacturers to ensure consistent dosing
- Risk: Low, but possible herb-drug interactions if on anticoagulants or NSAIDs

For stress and anxiety:

- Evidence: Ashwagandha reduces cortisol by 20-30% in multiple trials
- Mechanism: Stress hormone modulation through withanolide compounds
- Dose: 300-600 mg daily for 6-8 weeks
- Source: Standardized extracts (KSM-66, Sensoril are studied formulations)
- Risk: May interact with sedatives; not for pregnancy/lactation

For cognitive support:

- Evidence: Brahmi shows improved memory in some studies, though larger trials needed
- Mechanism: Neurotransmitter modulation, antioxidant effects
- Dose: 300 mg daily of standardized bacosides
- Source: Standardized extracts ensuring consistent alkaloid content
- Risk: Minimal documented toxicity

The pattern: evidence-based herb use combines traditional wisdom with modern standardization, dosing, and safety monitoring.

Synthesis: The Future of Ayurveda in Evidence-Based Medicine.

For India's healthcare future, Ayurveda's role is increasingly clear:

NOT a replacement for evidence-based medicine in acute conditions, surgery, or infectious disease.

BUT excellent for:

- Chronic disease prevention
- Inflammation management
- Stress and anxiety reduction

- Immune support
- Quality of life and long-term health maintenance
- Personalized health approaches based on individual constitution

The Integration Framework

The future isn't Ayurveda versus allopathy. It's integrated evidence-based medicine that respects traditional wisdom while demanding rigorous testing:

1. Fund rigorous clinical trials on promising Ayurvedic herbs using pharmaceutical-quality methodologies
2. Standardize production to ensure consistent phytochemical content
3. Implement quality control testing for heavy metals, microbial contamination, and potency
4. Document pharmacogenomics to identify which individuals benefit from specific herbs
5. Develop herb-drug interaction databases to prevent dangerous combinations
6. Train practitioners in evidence-based practice, not just traditional lore

Practical Actions for Young Indians

If you believe in Ayurveda:

- Ask practitioners for evidence, mechanism of action, and specific dosing
- Use standardized extracts from reputable manufacturers, not random market powders
- Combine with conventional medicine for serious conditions, not instead of
- Report herb use to conventional doctors to check for interactions

If you're skeptical:

- Recognize that lack of rigorous evidence isn't lack of effect; it's lack of funding for testing
- Acknowledge that your grandmother's turmeric milk has legitimate biochemistry, even if not pharmaceutical grade
- Consider low-risk, low-cost herbs as supplements to

conventional care, not replacements
- Demand standardization, transparency, and safety data from manufacturers

For India's development:

- Support research funding for Ayurvedic herb validation. India's 5,000-year-old pharmacopeia is an asset, not liability
- Invest in standardization infrastructure ensuring quality and consistency
- Create integrative medicine programs combining conventional and Ayurvedic practitioners
- Protect traditional knowledge from corporate biopiracy while promoting rigorous scientific validation

The Final Word (Or: Why Your Grandmother Was Right, Just Not For The Reasons She Thinks)

Your grandmother's turmeric milk works—not because mystical prana flows through curcumin molecules, not because her dosha balances every morning, but because curcumin is a potent anti-inflammatory compound that bioaccumulates with daily consumption, reducing systemic inflammation over months and years. The fact that it's traditionally consumed with black pepper means absorption optimization. The fact that she's shared this with family for decades means cultural meaning and stress reduction. These work together.

The Instagram supplement industry sells the same compounds but without the grandmother's consistency, community, and integration into daily life. The result: higher prices, lower adherence, and often suboptimal bioavailability.

Ayurveda isn't magic. It's not metaphysical energy channeling. It's sophisticated pharmacology that happens to predate the scientific method by 2,500 years. The herbs work—but we're only beginning to understand how, at which doses, for which individuals, with which mechanisms.

The bridge between traditional and evidence-based medicine isn't dismissing either. It's respecting grandmother's wisdom enough to test it rigorously, then integrating what works into modern healthcare.

Now go make turmeric milk exactly like your grandmother does—with black pepper, with fat (milk), with consistency. You're not just following tradition. You're optimizing pharmacokinetics.

Science validating grandmother wisdom is peak confirmation bias in the best way possible.

CHAPTER 9: SLEEP

The One Thing Indians Get Catastrophically Wrong (Or: Why Your All-Nighter Isn't A Personality Trait, It's Just Sleep Deprivation)

You're scrolling through LinkedIn at 3 AM—again—and your feed is flooded with performance gurus posting screenshots of their 4 AM wake-up times with captions: "While you sleep, champions are grinding! 💪 5 hours of sleep is all you need if you optimize! #Hustle #Grind #SelfMade." Meanwhile, your medical student cousin hasn't slept properly in three weeks and is running on caffeine, adrenaline, and spite. Your engineering roommate is bragging about pulling "only" three all-nighters this week instead of four, treating sleep deprivation like a badge of honor. Your mother is calling to ask why you look so tired, suggesting you "sleep better," as if sleep quality were a choice rather than a biological imperative.

Here's what neuroscience says: You're all collectively damaging your brains, and the sleep-is-for-weak-people culture is destroying Indian youth's cognitive performance, emotional regulation, and long-term health. A study of 72 Indian MBBS students tracked over 12 weeks found that as sleep duration declined from 6.8 ± 0.9 hours to 5.9 ± 1.1 hours, cognitive performance deteriorated measurably—reaction time worsened ($p < 0.001$), working memory declined ($p = 0.002$), and executive function degraded ($p < 0.001$). Academic performance showed a significant positive correlation with sleep duration ($r = 0.43$, p

= 0.001).

Translation: your all-nighter isn't making you smarter. It's literally shrinking your cognitive capacity. You're voluntarily reducing your own intellectual functioning while telling yourself it's ambition.

Let's talk about why your brain needs sleep more than it needs your LinkedIn posts.

The Neuroscience of Sleep (Or: Why Your Brain Has a Garbage Disposal That Only Works When You're Unconscious)

Sleep isn't a luxury. It's not downtime. It's active biological processing where your brain literally performs maintenance tasks impossible during wakefulness. Understanding sleep requires understanding two competing systems constantly negotiating with each other: the homeostatic drive and the circadian rhythm.

The Two-Process Model: Your Brain's Internal Schedule

Your sleep-wake cycle is governed by what neuroscientists call the "two-process model," developed by sleep researcher Borbély decades ago and still the most accurate framework we have:

Process S (Homeostatic Drive): This is your brain's sleep debt accumulator. The longer you stay awake, the more adenosine—a neurotransmitter byproduct of brain activity—accumulates in your brain. Think of adenosine as biological sediment that builds up throughout wakefulness. As adenosine increases, it activates sleep-promoting regions like the ventrolateral preoptic area (VLPO) and median preoptic nucleus (MnPO) in your hypothalamus. These regions produce GABA (gamma-aminobutyric acid), which inhibits wake-promoting neurons. Your brain is literally sending signals: "I need to shut down now."

When you sleep, adenosine decreases, clearing the neurochemical pressure. This is why sleep deprivation doesn't get "easier"—your adenosine keeps accumulating, increasing pressure for sleep.

Process C (Circadian Drive): Your circadian rhythm is a roughly 24-hour biological clock controlled by the suprachiasmatic nucleus (SCN) in your hypothalamus. This master clock is synchronized by light exposure—your eyes contain special photosensitive cells that send information about light/darkness to the SCN. During the day, your SCN inhibits melatonin (the sleep hormone) production. As evening approaches and light dims, melatonin increases, promoting sleepiness.

The interaction: You only sleep well when both Process S and Process C align. If it's your biological night (high melatonin, high adenosine) but you're staring at a bright phone screen (suppressing melatonin), you experience sleep tension—you need sleep but can't fall asleep.

Your night-shift engineer cousin isn't failing to sleep because of weak willpower. His Process C is inverted (his circadian clock is out of phase), while his Process S is paradoxically low during her biological day (when adenosine naturally decreases) and high during her biological night (when it's physiologically difficult to sleep). He's fighting his brain's fundamental operating system.

Sleep Architecture: The Sacred 90-Minute Cycle

Sleep isn't uniform. It's a cyclical alternation between two fundamentally different states:

NREM Sleep (Non-Rapid Eye Movement): Comprises ~75-80% of your night and progresses through three stages:

- N1 (Light Sleep): Transition stage, lasting minutes. This is when you're falling asleep and can be easily awakened.
- N2 (Light Sleep): Comprises 45-55% of total sleep. Your brain shows distinctive K-complexes and sleep spindles on EEG—electrical patterns associated with memory consolidation.
- N3 (Deep Sleep/Slow-Wave Sleep): The most restorative stage. Your brain shows slow-wave activity (delta waves on EEG) and is essentially "offline" for conscious awareness. This is when your body undergoes maximum physical restoration, growth hormone secretion peaks, and cellular repair accelerates. Unfortunately, N3 decreases linearly by approximately 2% per decade of life—a 10-year-old gets more deep sleep than a 30-year-old than a 50-year-old.

REM Sleep (Rapid Eye Movement): Comprises ~20-25% of your night, characterized by:

- Rapid eye movements (hence the name)
- Dreams (the most vivid, narratively complex dreams occur here)
- Temporary muscle paralysis (except your diaphragm, so you can breathe)
- High brain activity resembling wakefulness

REM sleep is crucial for memory consolidation (particularly emotional and procedural memories), creativity, mood regulation, and brain development.

The 90-Minute Cycle: These stages cycle repeatedly through the night in roughly 90-minute intervals (hence "ultradian rhythm"). Your first cycle might be 90 minutes of N1→N2→N3→brief REM. Your second cycle might extend REM. By your fifth cycle (8 hours later), you're spending 40+ minutes in REM and minimal time in N3.

This is why the last 2-3 hours of sleep matter disproportionately—that's when you get the most REM sleep. Cutting sleep short doesn't proportionally reduce total sleep time; it *catastrophically* reduces REM sleep, impairing emotional regulation, memory consolidation, and creativity.

The Brain's Garbage Disposal: The Glymphatic System

Here's where sleep gets genuinely fascinating. A 2023 discovery revealed that your brain has a literal waste-removal system—the glymphatic system—that activates primarily during sleep.

During wakefulness, your brain cells don't shrink much. During sleep, they shrink by approximately 60%, creating larger interstitial space. Cerebrospinal fluid (CSF) flows through this expanded space, washing away metabolic waste products like amyloid-beta and tau proteins—the proteins that accumulate in Alzheimer's disease.

Sleep deprivation impairs this glymphatic clearance. Wake continuously, and metabolic waste accumulates in your brain. Do this chronically (as millions of Indian students and professionals do), and you're potentially accelerating neurodegeneration.

This isn't speculative. Sleep deprivation has been linked to increased risk of Alzheimer's disease, Parkinson's disease, and cognitive decline.

Blue Light and Melatonin Suppression: Why Your Phone Is Your Enemy

This is the mechanism destroying Indian students' sleep: blue light from screens suppresses melatonin production.

Blue light (wavelengths 380-495 nm) triggers special photosensitive cells in your retina called intrinsically photosensitive retinal ganglion cells (ipRGCs), which contain the photopigment melanopsin. These cells send direct signals to your SCN, essentially telling it: "It's daytime!". This delays melatonin release and advances your circadian clock.

A landmark 2015 PNAS study found that reading an iPad or similar light-emitting device for 2 hours before sleep:

- Suppressed melatonin by 20-25%
- Delayed sleep onset by 10+ minutes
- Reduced REM sleep duration

More recent research (2025) found that daily screen use was associated with later bedtimes and approximately 50 minutes less sleep per week—roughly 4 hours lost monthly from a single behavioral change.

For Indian college students sleeping 5-6 hours already (not the recommended 7-9 hours), losing 50 minutes weekly through screen time creates chronic sleep debt.

The brutal part: even if you use blue light filters, dark mode, or reduce brightness, screens still disrupt sleep through cognitive stimulation and circadian phase delays. Answering emails, scrolling Instagram, or watching YouTube before bed keeps your brain engaged and aroused.

Real-World Applications: From Medical Students to Software Engineers

The Indian Sleep Crisis: Quantifying the Disaster

College students: 95.3% of Indian college students sleep fewer than the recommended 7-8 hours. A 2025 study found that college students with chronic sleep deprivation showed progressive cognitive decline—reaction time worsened ($p < 0.001$), working memory declined ($p = 0.002$), and executive function deteriorated ($p < 0.001$).

Medical students: The situation is apocalyptic. Indian MBBS students in one study averaged 5.9 ± 1.1 hours nightly. Over 12 weeks of tracking, those sleeping less than 6 hours showed academic performance decline correlated with sleep deprivation ($\beta = +2.78$, $p = 0.003$)—meaning each additional hour of sleep was associated with 2.78-point academic score improvement.

Engineering students: Anecdotal reports suggest 4-5 hours average, with many treating all-nighters as normal. The cumulative cognitive impact is staggering.

Economic implications: Sleep deprivation costs India an estimated $55 billion annually in lost productivity—roughly 1.4% of GDP. This excludes healthcare costs from sleep-deprivation-related diseases.

The Neuroscience Behind Cognitive Decline

What specifically deteriorates with sleep deprivation? Multiple domains measured in Indian studies:

Reaction Time: 24-hour sleep deprivation increased choice reaction time from 373.9 ± 63.5 ms to 435.7 ± 80.4 ms ($p = 0.01$). That's a 16.5% slowdown in neural processing speed—catastrophic for programming, surgery, or any cognitively demanding task.

Working Memory: Sleep-deprived students showed declined performance on digit span tests (105.4 ± 8.3 to 98.6 ± 17.9, $p = 0.03$). Your ability to hold information temporarily (needed for problem-solving, comprehension, focus) deteriorates measurably.

Executive Function: The Stroop test (measuring cognitive control and inhibitory function) showed progressive deterioration with sleep debt. You become impulsive, make worse decisions, struggle with task switching.

Attention and Concentration: Self-reported distractibility, forgetfulness, and "false triggering" (acting on autopilot incorrectly) all increased with sleep deprivation. You're not just slower—you're less accurate.

Emotional Regulation: Sleep deprivation impairs prefrontal-amygdala connectivity, meaning your rational brain loses control over your emotional brain. You become irritable, reactive, anxious, and emotionally unstable. Your cousin's aggressive behavior during exam season isn't personality—it's sleep deprivation creating neurological dysregulation.

Startup and Corporate Sleep Culture

Indian startups glorify sleep deprivation as hustle culture. Founders post about 4-5 hour sleep schedules like it's a competitive advantage. Neuroscience suggests they're literally reducing their own cognitive performance while congratulating themselves.

Research on startup founders shows that those prioritizing 7+ hours of sleep reported:

- Better decision-making (sleep improves prefrontal function)
- Increased creativity (REM sleep consolidates novel connections)
- Lower burnout (sleep restores emotional resilience)
- Better health (fewer sick days, lower disease risk)

Yet the culture persists. This is partly founder mythology (successful people slept little, so little sleep = success) and partly genuine misunderstanding of sleep physiology.

Critical Analysis: Debunking Sleep Myths

Myth 1: "You Can Adapt to 5 Hours of Sleep If You 'Optimize'"

No. You cannot adapt. Your brain requires sleep architecture (NREM → REM cycles) that requires time. Cutting sleep from 8 to 5 hours doesn't proportionally reduce your rest needs—it eliminates 40+ minutes of REM sleep per night.

Chronic sleep deprivation creates a sleep debt that accumulates daily. People chronically sleeping 5 hours show progressive cognitive decline, not plateau. Your brain doesn't "adapt"—it slowly deteriorates under constant adenosine pressure.

Myth 2: "Caffeine Replaces Sleep"

Caffeine masks fatigue but doesn't perform sleep's functions. Caffeine blocks adenosine receptors, preventing your brain from "sensing" adenosine accumulation. You feel alert while your brain accumulates unprocessed metabolic waste and skips memory consolidation, glymphatic clearance, and cellular repair.

Sleep debt accumulated despite caffeine still requires repayment through actual sleep.

Myth 3: "Weekday Sleep Deprivation Can Be Recovered on Weekends"

Partially true but with caveats:

- You can recover REM and NREM sleep partially on weekends
- But circadian disruption persists—your circadian clock can't completely resynchronize in one weekend
- Monday morning jet lag (your circadian misalignment) reduces cognitive performance despite weekend sleep recovery
- Chronic weekend catch-up creates "social jetlag"—your circadian clock is perpetually misaligned to your social schedule

Continuous irregular sleep (5 hours weekdays, 9 hours weekends) is worse than consistent 7-hour sleep nightly.

Myth 4: "Melatonin Supplements Substitute for Sleep"

Melatonin is a chronobiotic—it resets your circadian clock timing—but doesn't replace sleep's restoration functions. Melatonin might help you fall asleep if your circadian timing is disrupted, but it doesn't induce the full 90-minute sleep cycles your brain requires.

Taking a melatonin pill then forcing yourself to sleep-deprive isn't sleep. It's using a biological tool inefficiently.

Myth 5: "Short Sleepers Are Genetically Superior"

Some individuals have genetic variants producing shorter sleep needs (naturally needing 5-6 hours). These are exceptionally rare—probably <1-2% of the population. You're probably not one of them.

Claiming to be a "natural short sleeper" while showing cognitive impairment is statistical self-deception.

How Western Sleep Research Doesn't Fully Apply to India

Most sleep research comes from temperate zones with stable light cycles and air conditioning. India presents different challenges:

1. Heat and humidity: Indian summers disrupt sleep through thermoregulation challenges. AC helps but creates dependency.
2. Noise pollution: Urban India's constant noise (traffic, construction, neighbors) prevents deep sleep despite circadian alignment.
3. Irregular work/study schedules: Shift work, exams, and startup culture create non-24-hour schedules incompatible with circadian alignment.
4. Social jetlag: Large circadian-work schedule misalignment in India creates perpetual circadian disruption.

Western "optimize sleep with blue light filters" advice ignores that Delhi's sleep problem is heat, noise, and stress—not just screens.

The Thought Experiment: The Sleep Debt Accumulator

Imagine your brain has a sleep debt account. Each hour of sleep you need but don't get creates a debt. Unlike financial debt, sleep debt can't be ignored.

Scenario: You need 8 hours nightly but sleep 6 hours. Daily deficit: 2 hours. Over a week: 14 hours accumulated. Over a month: 60 hours. Over a year: 730 hours ≈ 30 days of continuous sleep debt.

This debt doesn't disappear. Your adenosine keeps accumulating. Your glymphatic system can't clear metabolic waste fully. Your REM sleep quota goes unpaid.

By year-end, you're functioning as if you lost an entire month of sleep—and you did.

A Simple 2-Week Sleep Optimization Experiment

Week 1 - Baseline:

- Sleep naturally (no alarms if possible) for 3 nights, tracking hours slept

- Avoid screens 1 hour before bed but don't force sleep discipline otherwise
- Track subjective focus, mood, reaction time (reaction speed to unexpected situations)

Week 2 - Intervention:

- Prioritize 8 hours nightly (adjust bedtime accordingly)
- No screens 1.5 hours before bed
- No caffeine after 2 PM
- Keep room temperature 18-20°C (optimal sleep temperature)
- Track same metrics

Observation: Most people report improved focus, reaction time, mood, and emotional regulation within 2 weeks. Some report it's "too much to prioritize."

That discomfort is your brain recovering from chronic sleep deprivation—you're not used to feeling well-rested.

Synthesis: Sleep as India's Most Underrated Resource

For a nation facing cognitive challenges—competitive exams, startup culture, intense academic pressure—sleep is free, unlimited, and massively effective. Yet it's systematically stigmatized.

The paradox: Indian culture simultaneously:

- Valorizes work ethic and all-nighters (Hustle Culture)
- Complains about declining cognitive performance and rising depression (Reality)
- Refuses to acknowledge that these are causally connected (Denial)

Sleep isn't laziness. It's the foundation of cognitive performance, emotional health, disease prevention, and long-term productivity.

Practical Actions for 2025

1. Calculate your sleep debt: How many hours below 8 do you sleep nightly? Over a month? A year? Seeing the accumulated total is jarring.

2. Protect your circadian rhythm: Consistent sleep schedule matters more than total hours. Going to bed at 10 PM nightly is better than irregular 11 PM/2 AM/midnight schedules.

3. Implement screen curfew: No screens 1.5 hours before bed. Yes, this is hard. Your sleep quality depends on it.

4. Optimize sleep environment: Cool (18-20°C), dark, quiet room. This is free/cheap and produces measurable sleep improvement.

5. Challenge hustle culture: Recognize that "sleeping only 5 hours" is self-imposed cognitive damage, not ambition. High performers sleep adequately—Steve Jobs prioritized sleep, as did LeBron James.

6. For India's future: Educational institutions should implement sleep hygiene programs. Medical schools, IITs, and startups should normalize 7-8 hour sleep as performance requirement, not weakness.

7. Mental health perspective: Sleep deprivation is a major contributor to anxiety and depression in Indian youth. Solving the sleep crisis potentially solves a significant mental health crisis.

The Final Word (Or: Why Your All-Nighter Is Literally Making You Stupid)

Sleep isn't rest. It's active biological processing where your brain performs maintenance impossible during wakefulness—memory consolidation, metabolic waste clearance, emotional regulation, cellular repair.

Your all-nighter doesn't make you hardworking. It makes your cognitive performance measurably worse—slower reaction time, impaired working memory, degraded executive function, reduced creativity, emotional dysregulation. You're sacrificing tomorrow's cognitive performance for today's study hours.

The sleep-culture mythology—that successful people sleep little and sacrifice rest for ambition—confuses correlation with causation. Successful people didn't sleep little *because* they were successful. They succeeded *despite* inadequate sleep. If they'd optimized sleep, they'd likely be even more successful.

For Indian youth facing incredible academic and professional pressure, sleep is your superpower. Not because it feels good (though it does), but because it's literally foundational to cognitive performance, emotional health, and long-term productivity.

Now stop reading, set your phone down, turn off your lights, and—for once—give your brain what it actually needs.

Your circadian rhythm has been waiting all day for this moment.

Sleep isn't weakness. It's the only reason your brain works.

CHAPTER 10: HUMAN CONNECTION

The Free Drug No One's Taking (Or: Why Your Loneliness Is Literally Aging Your Arteries)

You're scrolling through Instagram at 2 AM in your Bangalore apartment, surrounded by 8 million people, yet feeling utterly alone. Your Instagram stories show you at parties, weddings, and networking events—the picture of social butterfly-dom. Meanwhile, 47% of young adults in urban India report feelings of loneliness despite living in the most connected cities on Earth. You've got 2,000 Instagram followers but nobody to call at 3 AM when you're spiraling. Your group chat from engineering college is active daily with memes, yet you haven't had a genuine conversation with any of those people in months. You're "friends" with 500 people but feel fundamentally disconnected from all of them.

Here's what science says about this disconnection: Loneliness is not just an emotional state. It's a biological catastrophe that ages your cardiovascular system at an accelerated rate, increases your risk of premature death by 29%, and kills more people annually than COVID-19 did at its peak. The WHO estimates loneliness causes 871,000 deaths annually—roughly one death every 36 seconds.

Young adults experiencing loneliness are showing early markers of arterial stiffness—the kind of vascular damage you'd expect in people decades older. Your Instagram likes cannot fix this. Your network size cannot fix this. Only actual human connection can—and we're collectively failing spectacularly at it.

Let's talk about why your brain literally needs other humans to function, and what happens when you don't get them.

The Neuroscience of Connection (Or: Why Evolution Designed You as a Social Creature, Not an Instagram Account)

Humans are not meant to be individuals. Evolutionarily, solitary humans died quickly. In groups, they survived. This isn't poetic philosophy—it's written into your neurobiology at the deepest levels.

Mirror Neurons: The Biological Empathy Mechanism

When you watch someone touch a hot stove, your brain's somatosensory cortex activates as if *you* touched it. When you see someone smile, your facial muscles micro-contract as if you were smiling. This is the mirror neuron system—a network of neurons that fire both when you perform an action and when you observe someone else performing it.

Discovered in primates in the 1990s by Italian neuroscientist Vittorio Rizzolatti, mirror neurons are the neural basis of empathy, imitation, and social learning. They're why watching others creates understanding without explicit teaching. They're why watching someone in pain activates your pain centers. They're why seeing someone cry makes you sad.

More importantly, mirror neurons trigger oxytocin release—the neurochemical at the foundation of all social bonding. When your mirror neurons fire in response to someone else's experience, they activate brain regions that release oxytocin, creating a cascade of neurobiological events: decreased anxiety, increased trust, enhanced empathy, improved emotional regulation.

Think of mirror neurons as your brain's social synchronization mechanism. When you're with people, your brains literally harmonize. When you're isolated, there's nobody to synchronize with, and your neurochemistry drifts into dysregulation.

Oxytocin: The Social Glue Hormone

Oxytocin is often called the "love hormone" or "cuddle chemical," which is reductive but not entirely wrong. This neuropeptide does two critical things:

1. Creates Social Attachment: Oxytocin levels increase when you hug someone, have sex, eat with others, or engage in cooperative activities. It literally makes social interaction feel rewarding.

2. Reduces Threat Response: Oxytocin simultaneously decreases amygdala (fear center) activation and reduces cortisol (stress hormone) production. Social connection literally calms your nervous system.

The mechanism: when you're with trusted people, mirror neurons fire, oxytocin releases, your amygdala quiet down, your cortisol drops, and you feel safe. Your cardiovascular system relaxes, your blood pressure normalizes, your inflammatory markers decrease.

Conversely, when you're chronically isolated, your amygdala stays vigilant, cortisol stays elevated, your nervous system remains in mild fight-or-flight mode. Your body interprets loneliness as threat, activating the same stress response mechanisms that would activate if you were physically endangered.

Chronic low-grade threat response = chronic inflammation = accelerated aging of your cardiovascular system.

The Attachment System: Your Brain's Survival Expectation

From infancy, your brain develops an attachment system—a neurobiological framework expecting consistent, reliable relationships. When this expectation is met, your brain receives a signal: "You're safe. You belong. Your needs matter.". When it's not met, your brain receives: "You're unsafe. You don't belong. Your survival is at risk.".

This isn't optional or psychological in nature. It's a hardwired survival system. And it operates continuously throughout your life, not just childhood.

Modern urban isolation creates a peculiar situation: you're physically surrounded by millions of people, yet your attachment system receives zero signals of secure connection. You have social media "friends" who don't know you exist. You have group chats replacing genuine conversation. You have surface-level networking replacing deep friendship.

Your brain doesn't distinguish between "alone" and "lonely among millions." It just registers: "Attachment system not satisfied. Threat response activated.".

The Cardiovascular Consequences: Loneliness Ages Your Arteries

This is where it gets physiologically terrifying. A 2024 study examining 66 young adults (average age 22.7 years) found that higher loneliness was associated with shorter pulse transit time (PTT) after controlling for depression and anxiety. Shorter PTT indicates arterial stiffness—reduced elastic compliance of arteries. This is vascular damage you'd normally see in people decades older.

Researchers were alarmed: "These findings indicate that young adults experiencing higher levels of loneliness may already be exhibiting signs of vascular dysfunction or damage, evident as early as in their twenties".

The mechanism:

- Loneliness activates chronic stress response
- Elevated cortisol triggers systemic inflammation
- Inflammatory markers (IL-6, TNF-α, CRP) increase
- Endothelial dysfunction develops (arterial lining damaged)
- Arterial stiffness increases
- Blood pressure variability worsens
- Plaque formation accelerates
- Cardiovascular disease risk increases

The statistics are stark:

- Loneliness increases heart disease risk by 29%
- Loneliness increases stroke risk by 32%
- A 2025 systematic review of 13 studies with 63,978 participants found 43% increased risk of major adverse cardiovascular events (MACE) in isolated individuals
- Socially isolated individuals show higher mortality rates even after controlling for other risk factors

Real-World Applications: India's Loneliness Epidemic

The Urban Paradox: Connected Yet Alone

Indian cities are paradoxes. Mumbai has 20+ million people in crushing density. Delhi's metropolitan area approaches 30 million. Yet loneliness is skyrocketing.

Contributing factors specific to Indian context:

1. Migration and Rootlessness: Young professionals move to cities for careers, leaving family and childhood friends. They're physically alone despite urban density.

2. Hierarchical Workplace Culture: Indian corporate culture is often hierarchical and formal, discouraging genuine peer connection. You have colleagues, not friends.

3. Cultural Transition: Traditional Indian communities had built-in social structures (extended family, neighborhood connection, religious community). Urban nuclear families lack these.

4. Technology Replacing Touch: WhatsApp and Instagram replace physical presence, creating illusion of connection without actual connection.

5. Startup Culture Isolationism: The "hustle" mentality creates work-obsessed individuals sacrificing relationships for career advancement.

A 2025 study found that 47% of young adults in urban India report feelings of loneliness, with highest rates in metros (Mumbai, Delhi, Bangalore). Notably, frequency of social media use showed non-linear relationship with loneliness—people with moderate social media use showed lowest loneliness, while heavy users (>4 hours daily) showed rates comparable to isolated individuals.

Economic Impact: Loneliness Is Costing India Billions

Loneliness's economic impact in India is substantial but poorly quantified:

Healthcare costs: Lonely individuals show higher hospitalization rates, emergency department visits, and chronic disease management costs. A lonely person has 40% higher healthcare utilization.

Productivity loss: Lonely employees show decreased cognitive performance, lower engagement, higher absenteeism. An isolated team member reduces team collaboration and output.

Turnover: Lonely employees are more likely to leave organizations, creating recruitment/training costs.

Mental health burden: 73% of studies examining social isolation found increased depression and anxiety. Depression creates additional healthcare and productivity costs.

Extrapolating globally (where loneliness is estimated to cost $406 billion annually), India's costs likely exceed $10-15 billion annually.

Social Media's Complicated Relationship with Connection

Ironically, India's most connected people (heavy social media users) report higher loneliness. Why?:

Quality vs. Quantity: 2,000 Instagram followers ≠ genuine connection. Likes and comments don't satisfy attachment system needs.

Social Comparison: Seeing others' highlight reels creates inadequacy feelings and isolation rather than connection.

Performative Connection: Posting instead of calling. Commenting instead of conferencing. Texting instead of talking.

Algorithm Optimization: Social media algorithms show you content that engages (often negative, anxiety-inducing content), not content that connects.

However, positive interactions on social media do correlate with lower loneliness. A 2016 systematic review found that genuine social support and positive interactions on SNSs were associated with lower depression and anxiety. The distinction: supportive, genuine connection matters; performative, comparative scrolling worsens mental health.

Critical Analysis: Debunking Connection Myths

Myth 1: "Introversion Means You Don't Need Connection"

Introversion describes how you recharge energy (alone vs. social), not how much connection you need. Introverts require less *frequent* social interaction and recover from it faster, but they still require meaningful connection.

An isolated introvert is still experiencing loneliness, just with different social recovery patterns. "I'm introverted so I'm happy alone" is self-deception masking loneliness.

Myth 2: "Online Connection Is As Good As In-Person Connection"

No. Online connection activates mirror neuron systems less intensely than in-person interaction. Video calls activate more than text-only communication, but less than physical presence.

The oxytocin release from a Zoom call is measurably lower than from an in-person hug. Technology can supplement connection but cannot replace it.

Myth 3: "Quality Over Quantity—You Only Need A Few Friends"

Partially true with a dangerous caveat. Yes, depth matters more than number. But "deep connection with one person" doesn't fully satisfy the attachment system if that person is unavailable.

You need both depth (genuine understanding) AND reliability (consistent availability). A best friend in another country creating deep connection but zero physical contact may not satisfy attachment system needs.

Myth 4: "Loneliness Is Just Sadness"

Loneliness is a specific neurobiological state different from depression. You can be lonely in a crowd. You can be content alone (solitude). Loneliness specifically represents disconnection from desired connection.

The distinction matters because treatment differs. Depression requires different interventions than loneliness.

Myth 5: "You'll Outgrow Loneliness As You Get Older"

False. Loneliness remains stable across lifespan, though risk factors change. Young adults are less lonely than elderly in some contexts, yet young adult loneliness has increased substantially post-2015.

The neurobiological need for connection doesn't diminish with age—if anything, it intensifies as social networks shrink.

How Western Research Doesn't Fully Apply to Indian Context

Most social connection research comes from individualistic Western cultures emphasizing friend-groups and peer relationships. India's cultural context differs:

1. Extended Family: Historically provided built-in attachment relationships. Urban nuclear families lack this, creating new loneliness.

2. Caste/Community: Traditional vertical relationships (elder-younger) differ from horizontal peer relationships Western research emphasizes.

3. Hierarchical Relationships: Indian professional culture emphasizes hierarchy over peer friendship, creating different connection patterns.

4. Privacy Norms: Indian culture traditionally emphasized family privacy over friend-groups, now creating mismatch between traditional expectations and modern urban isolation.

Western "join clubs, make friends" advice ignores that Indian professionals work 12-hour days with hierarchical structures discouraging peer friendship.

The Thought Experiment: Your Loneliness Balance Sheet

Imagine loneliness as a bank account. Connection deposits make positive balance. Isolation withdrawals create deficit.

Deposits:

- In-person time with trusted people: +5 units

- Video call with close friend: +2 units
- Group activity/shared experience: +3 units
- Meaningful one-on-one conversation: +4 units

Withdrawals:

- Day alone: -1 unit
- Rejection or conflict: -3 units
- Watching others' social success: -2 units
- Isolated days/weeks: -5 per week

Your attachment system maintains a running balance. Negative balance (more withdrawals than deposits) = loneliness = stress activation = arterial damage.

Someone working 12 hours daily with 2-hour commute, living alone, making deposits of (occasional) video calls while experiencing weekly withdrawals of isolation is running a devastating deficit.

The calculation is individual but biological reality is universal: sustained negative balance harms your cardiovascular system.

A Simple Weekly Connection Audit

Track your week:

Genuine connection time: Minutes of conversation where someone actually knows you
Passive social media: Minutes scrolling, liking, but not connecting
Alone time: Hours without social contact
Planned connection: Time scheduled with specific people

Most isolated individuals show [high passive social media] + [high alone time] + [low genuine connection] + [zero planned connection].

The intervention: inverse the ratio. Reduce passive scrolling. Increase planned, genuine connection. Replace some alone time with structured social activity.

Synthesis: Connection as India's Most Underrated Resource

For a society prioritizing productivity, wealth accumulation, and individual achievement, connection is systematically devalued. "Stop socializing, focus on your career" is culturally reinforced. "Don't waste time on relationships" is the startup motto.

Yet the evidence is overwhelming: social connection is the strongest modifiable factor protecting against depression and cardiovascular disease. A single study analyzing data from 100,000+ people found that social connection was the strongest protective factor against depression—stronger than exercise, diet, sleep, or any other modifiable factor.

The irony: the one factor most protective of health is systematically sacrificed for factors less protective.

Practical Actions for 2025

1. Audit your connection: Track genuine connection time this week. Be honest about isolation levels.

2. Plan connection intentionally: Don't wait for it to happen. Schedule video calls with family. Join groups. Make friend time as mandatory as work meetings.

3. Distinguish between presence and connection: Sitting in the same room scrolling phones isn't connection. Actual conversation is.

4. Reduce parasocial relationships: Instagram followers aren't friends. YouTube channels aren't connection.

5. Find your community: Whether religious community, hobby groups, professional networks, or neighborhood—find your "tribe".

6. Prioritize depth over breadth: One genuine friend beats 500 acquaintances.

7. For India's development: Workplace cultures should encourage genuine peer connection, not just hierarchy. Cities should create spaces fostering community. Educational institutions should teach connection skills alongside STEM.

The Final Word (Or: Why Your Loneliness Is Literally Killing You, But It Doesn't Have To)

Evolution designed you for connection. Your mirror neurons, oxytocin system, and attachment architecture all evolved because solitary humans died, group humans survived.

Modernity created a situation where you can be surrounded by millions yet utterly alone—physically proximate, neurobiologically isolated.

The science is unequivocal: loneliness damages your cardiovascular system, increases depression and anxiety risk, and kills you prematurely. Not through sadness or psychological mechanisms alone, but through measurable biological pathways: chronic stress activation, systemic inflammation, arterial stiffening, immune dysregulation.

The pharmaceutical industry cannot fix this. No supplement, medication, or health optimization hack replaces genuine human connection. Your body doesn't care how many calories you counted or sleep hours you tracked. It cares whether you felt safe, understood, and valued by other humans.

For young Indians collectively sacrificing relationships for career advancement, here's the uncomfortable truth: your highest professional achievement means nothing if you arrive at it isolated and neurologically dysregulated.

The good news: connection is free. It requires no money, no special skills, no optimization. It requires only intention and time. An hour genuinely conversing with someone who cares about you activates all the protective neurobiological mechanisms that expensive wellness interventions try to simulate.

Now put this down. Call someone. Not to accomplish something. Not to network. Just to connect. Your arteries will thank you.

Loneliness is the most expensive health condition because it costs you your health.

CHAPTER 11: KNOWLEDGE SHARING

The Free Multiplier That Breaks Every Economic Law (Or: Why Teaching Someone Actually Makes You Smarter)

Your 11 PM WhatsApp shows a junior engineer asking you a question about database optimization. Your first instinct is to ignore it—you're exhausted, you've already solved this problem, why should you spend your time explaining it? But you answer anyway. Twenty minutes later, you've not only explained it clearly but discovered three approaches you never considered before. And somehow, despite the mental effort, you feel more energized than when the day started.

Meanwhile, your colleague—hoarding technical knowledge, refusing to mentor juniors, gatekeeping expertise to maintain job security—faces layoffs when the company reorganizes. Your company promotes you to team lead. The irony: by giving away your knowledge, you became more valuable. By protecting yours, your colleague became disposable.

Here's what neuroscience says about this paradox: Teaching activates your brain's learning systems more intensely than learning itself. When you explain something to someone else, your prefrontal cortex, temporal regions, and memory consolidation networks activate simultaneously, creating neural pathways stronger than the original learning. You're not just sharing information. You're reorganizing your own neural architecture to make it transferable, which paradoxically makes it stronger for you.

The economic implication: knowledge is the only resource that grows when shared. Unlike money (finite), energy (depletes), or time (irreplaceable), knowledge multiplies. When you teach someone, you keep your knowledge *and* they gain it.

India's knowledge economy is built on pretending this isn't true. Young professionals hide expertise, companies hoard intellectual capital, educational systems treat knowledge as competitive advantage rather than collaborative multiplication.

Let's talk about why the most successful people are usually the best teachers, and what that reveals about how human brains actually work.

The Neuroscience of Teaching (Or: Why Your Brain Treats Explaining as a Computational Problem)

When you learn something, specific brain regions activate: hippocampus (memory formation), prefrontal cortex (executive function), temporal lobe (language processing). When you teach that same information, a different network activates—more regions, higher cognitive load, deeper processing.

The Knowledge Transfer Brain Network: More Complex Than Learning

Teaching triggers what neuroscientists call the functional brain network of knowledge transfer—a distributed network coordinating multiple regions:

1. The Mentalizing Network:

- Medial Prefrontal Cortex (mPFC): Processes understanding of the learner's perspective. You're not just transmitting information; you're simulating their confusion, adapting your explanation based on their mental model.
- Temporoparietal Junction (TPJ): Theory of mind—inferring what the learner understands and misunderstands.
- The function: These regions activate strongly when you're teaching because you're constantly modeling the student's understanding (or lack thereof).

2. The Executive Function Network:

- Lateral Prefrontal Cortex (LPFC): Working memory, organizing information logically.
- The function: When explaining, you're not reciting memorized information—you're organizing knowledge on-the-fly, identifying connections, highlighting relationships.

3. The Memory Consolidation Network:

- Default Mode Network (DMN): Integrates new information with existing knowledge.
- Hippocampus: Normally important for learning, but during teaching, cortical regions become more active—suggesting knowledge is being reorganized into more stable, integrated form.

The twist: When you teach, your brain works *harder* than when you learn passively. Functional connectivity increases. Brain regions that weren't activated during passive learning now coordinate with each other.

Research quantifies this: Knowledge transfer activates brain regions with positive correlation coefficients (r = 0.545 to 0.623) with transfer performance. The brain expends genuine effort—measured as increased blood oxygenation, higher metabolic demand—to facilitate understanding in someone else.

Spaced Repetition and Teaching: The Consolidation Advantage

A key mechanism: teaching forces spaced learning on yourself.

Traditional spaced learning involves reviewing material at increasing intervals (see it day 1, review day 3, review week 2, review month 2). Each review strengthens memory through retrieval practice.

When you teach, you're *forced* to retrieve information, reorganize it for clarity, and defend it against questions. Each student interaction is a retrieval practice session with highest difficulty level—explaining rather than just remembering.

A 2025 study found that spaced learning-induced neural integration (measured by brain network connectivity) predicted durable memory lasting 1 month and beyond. The mechanism: distributed neural networks, not hippocampal activity alone, predict long-term retention.

Translation: Teaching creates the optimal neurocognitive conditions for memory durability. You retain taught material longer than material you merely studied.

The Brain's Preference: Giving vs. Receiving

Here's the genuinely surprising finding: your brain shows stronger reward activation when giving knowledge than receiving it.

When you learn, your brain receives information—dopamine releases from expectation and satisfaction. When you teach, your brain solves a problem (how to communicate this clearly to this person)—dopamine releases from solving, planning, perspective-taking.

More importantly, giving knowledge activates mentalizing networks more than receiving it. Your brain treats teaching as a social-cognitive challenge requiring deeper processing than passive reception.

Studies show that people report greater satisfaction from helping someone understand a concept than from learning the concept themselves. This isn't emotional preference—it's reflecting genuine neural activation patterns.

The evolutionary logic: humans are fundamentally social creatures. Knowledge sharing was survival advantage—communities where individuals taught each other survived better than isolated individuals. Evolution optimized brains to experience teaching as rewarding.

Real-World Applications: From Classroom to Startup

The Indian Education Crisis: Teaching Is Treated as Burden, Not Optimization

India's educational system treats teaching as a resource drain rather than an asset multiplication strategy:

1. Teacher-Student Ratios: Massive classes (50-100 students per teacher) prevent individualized knowledge transfer. Teaching requires perspective-taking, which is cognitively impossible at scale.

2. Rote Learning Over Explanation: Students memorize answers rather

than explaining concepts. This eliminates the brain activation benefits of teaching.

3. Knowledge Gatekeeping: Competitive exam culture treats knowledge as scarce resource to be hoarded, not abundant resource to be shared.

4. Mentorship Absence: Junior professionals receive instruction but not mentorship. They're told answers but don't teach, missing cognitive benefits of knowledge reorganization.

The cost: students never activate the teaching-related brain networks, so they develop weak neural consolidation of learned material. They forget quickly and relearn inefficiently.

A brain-based teaching approach (incorporating explanation, peer teaching, socratic dialogue) increases academic achievement by 22-35% compared to traditional lecture-only methods.

The irony: Teaching others would improve students' own learning, yet the system structures education to *prevent* teaching among peers.

Corporate Knowledge Hoarding: The Economic Waste

Indian startups and companies systematically discourage knowledge sharing:

- Individual contributor model: Rewarding people for work output, not knowledge transfer. Rational economic actors hide knowledge to maintain irreplaceability.
- No mentorship infrastructure: Junior engineers learn through trial-error-web-search rather than from experienced colleagues. Knowledge dies with employees.
- Competitive rather than collaborative culture: Cross-team knowledge sharing is rare. Each team protects its technical approaches as competitive advantage.

The result: knowledge that should be team/organizational asset remains individual silos. When someone leaves, organizational knowledge evaporates.

Economic models show that organizations implementing knowledge-sharing infrastructure (mentorship programs, documented best practices, collaborative learning) show 15-25% higher productivity despite no increase in resource input.

The mystery: if knowledge sharing is so economically valuable, why isn't every organization doing it?

Answer: Knowledge sharing requires trust, psychological safety, and reciprocity norms that aren't automatically present in hierarchical organizations. Creating these cultures is hard work with delayed ROI, so most organizations don't bother.

Tech Enabling Knowledge Transfer: The Emerging Infrastructure

Indian edtech and corporate platforms are finally building knowledge-sharing infrastructure:

- Mentorship platforms: Connecting junior professionals with experienced mentors for structured learning
- Documentation systems: Making organizational knowledge accessible and updateable rather than scattered in individual emails
- Internal social networks: Creating spaces for peer-to-peer knowledge sharing with social proof (likes, comments, citations)
- Learning communities: Github communities, Stack Overflow, open-source projects enabling asynchronous teaching

These platforms create explicit reciprocity norms (people help because they expect future help), reduce transaction costs of teaching (no need to find mentee; platform matches), and create social incentives (recognition, reputation).

The impact: organizations and communities with robust knowledge-sharing infrastructure show measurably higher learning outcomes and innovation compared to isolated knowledge hoarding.

Critical Analysis: Debunking Knowledge-Sharing Myths

Myth 1: "Teaching Takes Time Away From My Own Learning"

False. Teaching *is* learning—arguably the most intensive learning available. When you teach, you activate learning circuitry *plus* additional brain regions (mentalizing, executive function) not activated during passive study.

The misconception comes from conflating time input with cognitive benefit. Yes, teaching takes time. But that time produces stronger memory consolidation, more robust neural networks, and better transfer than equivalent study time.

An engineer spending 3 hours teaching database optimization to juniors learns it better than spending 3 hours re-reading documentation.

Myth 2: "If I Share My Knowledge, I Lose Competitive Advantage"

This assumes knowledge is finite and scarce. It isn't. When you share knowledge, you keep it *and* others gain it.

The "knowledge scarcity" strategy makes sense for proprietary algorithms or trade secrets. It doesn't make sense for conceptual knowledge, problem-solving approaches, or technical understanding.

Companies that hoard knowledge show higher turnover (people leave because they're not developing), lower innovation (siloed knowledge prevents combination), and higher hiring costs (must find external talent rather than developing internal talent).

Myth 3: "Only Experts Should Teach"

Completely false. Peer-to-peer teaching (where students teach each other) produces learning outcomes comparable to expert teaching. Often better, because peer-teachers recently struggled with concepts and remember confusion points experts forgot.

Additionally, peer teaching activates the teaching-related brain networks in both teacher and taught. Everyone benefits from the cognitive load and perspective-taking.

Indian engineering colleges restrict peer tutoring (assuming experts teach better). In reality, peer teaching would improve both peer-teachers' and peer-learners' understanding.

Myth 4: "Teaching is For Extroverts Who Like Public Speaking"

False. Teaching activates specific brain networks; extroversion is irrelevant. An introverted person explaining a concept one-on-one activates the same knowledge-transfer network as an extrovert lecturing a classroom.

One-on-one teaching might actually suit introverts better—same cognitive benefits without performance anxiety.

How Western Research Doesn't Apply to Indian Contexts

Most knowledge-sharing research comes from Western organizations emphasizing open communication and psychological safety.

India's hierarchical cultures, competitive academic environments, and job market that rewards individual achievement over team development create different incentive structures:

1. Hierarchy: Junior professionals can't teach seniors; the social structure prevents it.

2. Scarcity mentality: When jobs are scarce (especially in competitive fields), knowledge hoarding is rational—you can't be replaced if only you know.

3. Transience: High turnover in Indian startups means people don't invest in knowledge transfer (you might leave, why teach?)..

4. Exam culture: Schools train students to compete for grades, not collaborate through teaching.

These aren't individual failures—they're rational responses to structural incentives. Changing knowledge-sharing culture requires changing those incentives, which is organizationally difficult.

The Thought Experiment: Your Knowledge-Sharing Account

Imagine an organizational knowledge account: deposits are teaching/documentation, withdrawals are departures without handoff:

Organization A: Engineers teach juniors regularly, document

approaches, leave detailed documentation. Knowledge deposit rate exceeds employee turnover. Organizational knowledge grows annually despite 20% turnover.

Organization B: Engineers hoard knowledge, document minimally, provide no mentorship. Knowledge withdraws with departing employees. Each turnover loses engineering approaches, debugging methods, hard-won insights.

After 5 years:

- Org A: Robust knowledge base, reduced hiring burden (internal talent pipeline), lower training costs
- Org B: Perpetual rebuilding, high hiring costs, lost institutional knowledge

The paradox: Org A's apparent "time investment" in teaching produces net economic gain. Org B's apparent "efficiency" (no time wasted on teaching) produces net economic loss.

A Simple 2-Week Teaching Experiment

Pick one concept you know well. Commit to explaining it to 3-5 different people in different contexts:

Week 1:

- Explain to a peer in your field
- Explain to someone outside your field
- Write a detailed explanation for documentation
- Create a simple visual explaining the concept

Week 2:

- Reflect on how your understanding evolved
- Notice which explanations worked best
- Identify gaps in your own understanding revealed by teaching
- Track your confidence in the concept before/after

Most people report 20-30% deeper understanding after a week of active teaching compared to baseline.

This isn't magic—it's your brain consolidating knowledge through retrieval, organizing it logically, and integrating it across neural networks.

Synthesis: Knowledge Sharing as India's Most Underutilized Development Tool

For a developing nation competing in the global knowledge economy, India's knowledge-hoarding culture is economically catastrophic.

China invested in knowledge transfer infrastructure—mentorship programs, documentation systems, cross-company learning networks. Result: rapid innovation cycles, higher productivity growth.

India invested in gatekeeping—competitive exams, knowledge scarcity signaling, individual achievement emphasis. Result: brilliant individuals, fragmented organizations, slow innovation scaling.

The neuroscience is clear: teaching literally optimizes learning. Knowledge sharing multiplies organizational capacity. Mentorship develops talent at 1/10 the hiring cost.

Yet the culture systematically discourages all three.

Practical Actions for 2025

1. Become a mentor: Formally mentor 1-2 junior people. You'll improve your own expertise.

2. Document your knowledge: Write down approaches, lessons learned, debugging strategies. Future you and future colleagues will thank present you.

3. Teach openly: Present on topics you know, answer questions publicly (instead of via private DMs), create visible knowledge.

4. Join knowledge communities: Github, Stack Overflow, open-source projects, professional associations—spaces facilitating knowledge sharing.

5. Push organizational change: Advocate for mentorship infrastructure, documentation systems, internal knowledge-sharing platforms.

6. For managers: Design work rewarding knowledge transfer, not just

individual output. Create psychological safety enabling risk-taking and question-asking.

7. For educators: Replace lectures with peer teaching, Socratic dialogue, student-led explanations. Students learn better AND teach better when given opportunity.

The Final Word (Or: Why Teaching Is The Ultimate Self-Care)

The traditional framing of knowledge sharing as sacrifice—"I'm helping them but losing time"—completely inverts reality.

Teaching is optimal learning. It activates more brain regions than passive study, consolidates memory more robustly, produces stronger transfer to new contexts.

When you teach, you're not being altruistic at the expense of yourself. You're optimizing your own neural architecture.

The person who taught you database optimization wasn't sacrificing their learning. They were *achieving* the deepest possible learning through the act of explaining.

For India's future—competing globally, developing workforce, building sustainable growth—knowledge sharing isn't nice-to-have. It's foundational economic infrastructure.

Every junior engineer not mentored is engineering capacity lost. Every approach not documented is debugging effort wasted. Every engineer hoarding knowledge instead of teaching is optimizing for individual job security instead of organizational multiplication.

The countries succeeding aren't those with the smartest individuals. They're those with infrastructure and culture enabling knowledge multiplication—where each person's learning benefits from accumulated organizational wisdom.

Now close this and teach someone something. Not to help them (though you are). To optimize your own learning. To multiply your knowledge. To build the infrastructure your country desperately needs.

Your brain will handle the heavy lifting. It's literally designed for this.

Teaching isn't losing knowledge. It's crystallizing it into permanent architecture.

CHAPTER 12: SELFLESS SERVICE (SEVA)

The Free High That's Better Than Any Drug (Or: Why Your Brain Loves Helping Others Even When You Don't Think You Do)

Your Instagram story shows you at a charity fundraiser, hashtag #ServiceWithaSmile #BetterWorld #MakingaDifference. But between you and me, you spent the evening networking, watching others volunteer, and secretly calculating whether this would look good on your resume. Meanwhile, your grandmother spent the afternoon preparing meals for widows in her neighborhood—no hashtag, no recognition, no social media documentation. She didn't announce it. She just did it. And when you saw her after, she had an inexplicable lightness about her, despite her chronic arthritis pain.

Here's what neuroscience says about that: Your grandmother's brain just experienced a pharmacological event comparable to taking a mild opiate—without any of the addiction potential or overdose risk. Her nucleus accumbens (reward center) flooded with dopamine. Her body released endorphins (natural opioids) and oxytocin (the bonding hormone). Her stress hormones (cortisol, adrenaline) plummeted. And the cardiovascular benefits of her afternoon's service will protect her against heart disease more effectively than most medications.

Your Instagram performance produced zero of these benefits. Her authentic seva produced measurable neurochemical cascade.

Let's talk about why your brain is literally designed to experience euphoria from helping others, and why modern India—obsessed with personal achievement and individual success—is collectively depriving itself of this free medicine.

The Neuroscience of Altruism (Or: Why Your Brain Has a Reward System That Activates When You Sacrifice)

Evolution designed a bizarre neurobiological paradox: your brain's reward system activates most intensely not when you benefit yourself, but when you benefit others at cost to yourself. This seems irrational. It's actually survival genius.

The Brain's Reward Circuitry: More Than Just Dopamine

When you help someone, multiple brain regions activate simultaneously, creating a distinct neurological signature of altruism:

1. The Mesolimbic Pathway (Reward Circuit):

- Ventral Tegmental Area (VTA): The dopamine production hub. When you witness the positive impact of your help, your VTA floods dopamine into the nucleus accumbens.
- Nucleus Accumbens (NaCC): The pleasure center. Dopamine binding here creates the sensation of reward and satisfaction.
- The twist: This activation is strongest when your helping is *costly* to you—when you sacrifice time, money, or comfort. Pure monetary gain activates these regions mildly. Costly altruism activates them powerfully.

2. The Mentalizing Network:

- Medial Prefrontal Cortex (mPFC): Processes your understanding of others' mental states.
- Temporoparietal Junction (TPJ): Enables theory of mind—inferring what others are thinking/feeling.
- The mechanism: By understanding *why* someone needs help and *how* your action helps them, you activate these regions. More understanding = greater reward activation = deeper satisfaction.

3. The Emotional Salience Network:

- Anterior Cingulate Cortex (ACC): Processes emotional significance and pain/conflict monitoring.

- The function: When you see someone suffering and contemplate alleviating that suffering, your ACC lights up. When you successfully help, ACC activity decreases (pain resolved).

The integrated system: Understanding someone's need (mPFC/TPJ) → contemplating your action (ACC monitoring) → witnessing relief (dopamine release) → feeling satisfaction (NaCC activation) → motivation to help again (forward loop).

This creates positive feedback loop: help → feel good → want to help more → help more → feel better.

The Helper's High: More Than One Chemical

The colloquial "helper's high" is real, but it's not just dopamine. It's a cocktail of neurochemicals:

Endorphins: The body's natural opioids. Helping triggers endorphin release similar to how the body responds to light physical pain—it *hurts* a little (you're sacrificing), then releases endorphins (the pain feels good). This is why people describe helping as both effortful and profoundly satisfying.

Dopamine: Reward and motivation. The feeling of pleasure and the motivation to repeat behavior.

Oxytocin: The bonding hormone. Helping someone directly (not just donating money) releases oxytocin, creating feelings of connection, warmth, and prosocial motivation. This is why face-to-face volunteer work produces more intense feelings than anonymous donations.

Serotonin: Mood regulation. Acts of kindness increase serotonin, contributing to improved mood and self-worth.

Together, these create a neurochemical state subjectively experienced as warmth, satisfaction, purpose, and sometimes euphoria. The traditional term "helper's high" understates it—it's more like a gentle opiate high combined with mood elevation and emotional connection.

The Cardiovascular Magic: How Seva Actually Extends Your Life

Here's where it gets genuinely dramatic. A 2024 longitudinal study tracking 5,079 adults over 12 years (Health and Retirement Study) found:

Volunteering a moderate number of hours → 46% lower heart attack risk

High purpose in life + high-commitment volunteering → Even greater protection

The mechanism involves multiple pathways:

1. Behavioral improvements: Volunteers naturally adopt healthier behaviors—more physical activity, better diet, stress reduction. The volunteer activity itself provides physical activity and social engagement.
2. Stress hormone reduction: Chronic helping reduces baseline cortisol and adrenaline. Whereas chronic stress damages cardiovascular tissue, chronic altruism strengthens it.
3. Inflammatory marker reduction: Volunteers show lower IL-6, TNF-α, and other inflammatory markers associated with heart disease.
4. Social support: Volunteering creates community connection, which itself has documented cardiovascular benefits.

The result: volunteers show cardiovascular biomarkers comparable to people 10-15 years younger than their chronological age.

For context, a 46% reduction in heart attack risk is comparable to some medications. Yet it's free, has no side effects, and produces additional mental health benefits.

Real-World Applications: From Urban Alienation to Village Seva

The Indian Seva Crisis: Abundance Yet Isolation

India has a paradoxical relationship with seva. The cultural concept is ancient and embedded in Hindu, Buddhist, and Sikh traditions. Yet modern urban India is increasingly isolated and service-disconnected.

Contributing factors:

1. Urbanization and Nuclear Families: Traditional joint families and village communities had built-in seva structures—elder care, community support, mutual help. Nuclear urban families lack these.

2. Professionalization of Care: Elderly parents go to nursing homes. Community members are paid care workers. Mutual aid becomes commercial transaction.

3. Social Atomization: Urban professionals work 12+ hours with commutes, leaving zero energy for seva. The time cost of helping feels prohibitive.

4. Performative Volunteering: CSR (Corporate Social Responsibility) creates "checkbox" volunteering—one annual event for company image, not genuine service.

5. Wealth and Distance: Wealthier Indians increasingly isolate from lower-income communities through gated societies, private vehicles, and private services—reducing natural opportunities for service interaction.

The result: young urban Indians experience unprecedented seva deprivation despite living in communities that desperately need service.

The Economic Case for Seva: Impossible to Quantify, Crucial to Calculate

Volunteering's economic impact is massive but invisible because it's not monetized:

Healthcare savings: Volunteers show 46% lower cardiovascular disease risk, 22-32% lower disease risk generally. Extrapolating to India's volunteer-eligible population (urban professionals), reduced healthcare utilization saves potentially ₹10,000-50,000 crore annually.

Productivity gains: Volunteers report increased life satisfaction, decreased depression, better focus. The productivity difference is measurable but uncalculated.

Social cohesion benefits: Communities with high volunteering show lower crime, higher educational attainment, better mental health. Quantifying this is nearly impossible but economically massive.

Healthcare cost prevention: A person with clinical depression or cardiovascular disease creates enormous healthcare expenses. Volunteering prevents both.

The irony: investing in volunteering infrastructure (creating safe ways for professionals to serve, incorporating seva into workplace culture, building volunteer networks) would pay enormous returns through health benefits and community resilience—yet it's systematically underfunded.

Technology Enabling Seva: The Emerging Space

Indian startups are beginning to create volunteering infrastructure:

- Platforms like CauseIndia, Aashayein: Matching volunteers with opportunities, reducing friction to participation
- Corporate volunteering apps: Allowing employees to log volunteer hours, creating social proof and accountability
- Community skill-sharing: Online platforms connecting professionals (lawyers, doctors, engineers) with underserved communities for pro-bono service
- Impact measurement: Apps tracking volunteer contributions and demonstrating impact, activating the reward circuitry by showing results

The potential: removing friction to seva participation could dramatically increase volunteering, accessing neurobio logical benefits currently unavailable to isolated urban professionals.

Critical Analysis: Debunking Altruism Myths

Myth 1: "True Altruism Must Have Zero Benefit to the Helper"

This is philosophically seductive but neurobiologically inaccurate. Your brain evolved to experience reward from helping others *precisely because* that reward motivates future helping.

If helping provided zero benefit to the helper, humans wouldn't help—natural selection would select for non-helpers. Instead, humans evolved such that helping produces intense satisfaction.

So the "pure altruism" question is confused. When you experience helper's high, you're not being selfish—you're experiencing your evolutionary heritage. The satisfaction is the *mechanism* ensuring you help, not evidence that you're not truly altruistic.

Myth 2: "Volunteering Should Only Be About the Recipient's Benefit"

No. The giver's benefits are real and should be acknowledged. Recognizing these benefits doesn't diminish the service—it explains why service works as medicine.

Young Indians should volunteer partly *because* it benefits them—because their cardiovascular system needs it, their mental health needs it, their dopamine system needs it.

This isn't selfish. It's acknowledging that helping others *is* helping yourself.

Myth 3: "Anonymous Donations Are As Rewarding As Direct Service"

False. Brain activity differs significantly:

- Monetary donation: Modest nucleus accumbens activation, no mentalizing network involvement.
- Direct volunteer work: Intense activation across reward regions, strong mentalizing network involvement, high oxytocin release.

Why: Monetary donations are abstract. Direct service involves witnessing the recipient's gratitude, understanding their story, experiencing connection. More understanding = more activation = more reward.

For maximum neurobiological benefit, *face-to-face, personal service* matters more than financial contribution.

Myth 4: "Busy Professionals Can't Volunteer"

Logistically true (time constraints are real). Neurobiologically false—even modest volunteering produces measurable benefits.

The study finding: moderate-hours volunteering showed 46% heart attack risk reduction (comparable to high-commitment volunteering).

Translation: even occasional service produces major benefits.

For Indian professionals working 12-hour days, *some* volunteering (monthly service day, occasional mentoring) produces greater health benefits than zero volunteering.

How Western Research Doesn't Apply to India

Most volunteering research comes from developed nations with established volunteer infrastructure and cultural emphasis on individual volunteerism.

India's context differs critically:

1. Service as cultural expectation: Traditional seva is communal obligation, not individual choice. Rural India still operates this way.

2. Service infrastructure weakness: Formal volunteer organizations are limited. Much helping is informal (family obligation, neighborhood assistance).

3. Economic constraints: Many Indians lack free time for volunteering—they're economically surviving, not seeking fulfillment.

4. Caste and service: Traditional caste hierarchy complicated service relationships. Some service was mandatory, not optional.

Western "go volunteer and feel better" advice ignores that Indian service relationships are often obligatory (family elder care), constrained by economic desperation (no time), or complicated by social hierarchy.

Yet the neurobiology remains universal: authentic service activates reward circuitry regardless of context.

The Thought Experiment: Your Seva Account

Imagine your neurological health as a savings account, similar to financial accounts:

Deposits (service/altruistic behavior):

- Volunteering 1-2 hours weekly: +10 units dopamine/oxytocin
- Direct service (mentoring, helping neighbors): +15 units
- Anonymous donation: +3 units
- Financial contribution with no relational involvement: +1 unit

Withdrawals (isolation, self-focus):

- Isolated day: -2 units
- Self-focused work without service: -1 unit daily
- Chronic isolation: -5 units weekly

Your neurological account balance determines your cardiovascular health, mental health, and longevity.

Someone working in a high-paying job with zero service, living isolated in a gated apartment, making annual CSR donations but no personal service is running a devastating deficit. Someone earning less but embedded in community service shows neurological abundance.

The wealthy, isolated professional has both money and poverty—financial wealth, neurobiological poverty.

A Simple Weekly Seva Experiment

Week 1 - Baseline:

- Track your mood (1-10 scale) daily
- Track your energy levels
- Note any physical symptoms (aches, sleep quality, digestion)
- Record zero intentional service acts

Week 2 - Intervention:

- Commit to 2-4 hours of *direct* service (mentoring, community work, helping family with no expectation of return)
- Track same metrics
- Pay attention to mood shifts, energy changes, physical improvements

Expected observation: Most people report improved mood, better sleep, reduced muscle tension within one week.

This isn't placebo—it's your dopamine-oxytocin system responding to authentic service.

Synthesis: Seva as India's Most Underutilized Medicine

For a culture simultaneously drowning in cardiovascular disease, mental health crises, and social atomization, the solution is paradoxically free: authentic service.

India's healthcare system is overwhelmed. Mental health infrastructure is insufficient. Preventive medicine is underprioritized. Yet the most powerful preventive intervention—seva—remains culturally devalued in urban contexts.

A person volunteering 4 hours weekly receives cardiovascular benefits equivalent to consuming specific medications for years, yet experiences zero side effects and massive mental health improvements.

Yet we stigmatize time spent serving as "not productive" while celebrating time spent working toward individual gain.

Practical Actions for 2025

1. Reframe volunteering: It's not altruism requiring sacrifice. It's medicine—effective, free, and delivered through helping others.

2. Start locally: You don't need to join formal organizations. Mentor a younger person. Help elderly neighbors. Teach your skills to someone who needs them.

3. Make it direct: Face-to-face service activates your reward circuitry; anonymous donations don't. Prioritize relational service.

4. Measure impact: Track your mood, sleep, stress levels before and after 4 weeks of weekly service. You'll notice measurable improvements.

5. For employers: Incorporating volunteer opportunities into workplace culture isn't charity—it's employee health optimization. Employees who volunteer show better performance, lower burnout, reduced healthcare costs.

6. For India's development: Normalize seva as equally valuable to career advancement. Recognize that a person serving 10 hours weekly is healthier, more resilient, and more productive than someone grinding 60 hours with zero service.

7. Rebuild infrastructure: Create digital platforms, safe spaces, and organizational structures enabling people to serve, particularly in urban contexts where informal service is impossible.

The Final Word (Or: Why Your Grandmother Knows What Neuroscience Is Just Now Discovering)

Your grandmother didn't serve because neuroscience proved it was healthy. She served because her culture embedded seva in identity, her family structure required it, and ultimately—her biology rewarded it.

Modern neuroscience has validated what traditional cultures always knew: helping others isn't sacrifice. It's self-preservation cloaked in generosity.

The neurochemistry is simple: authentic service activates reward circuits, reduces stress hormones, strengthens cardiovascular system, elevates mood, creates purpose. These aren't spiritual benefits. These are measurable, biological consequences of helping others.

For young Indians collectively stressed, isolated, and depressed despite unprecedented wealth and connectivity, the solution isn't more apps, better salaries, or greater achievement. It's service—authentic, direct, relational helping of people in need.

The irony of modern India: we've built healthcare systems to treat cardiovascular disease, mental illness, and loneliness—conditions that authentic seva prevents. We spend thousands on mental health apps and cardiovascular medications when the most powerful intervention is free and available to anyone willing to help someone else.

Now close this chapter, identify someone who needs help (elderly neighbor, younger mentee, underserved community), and spend a few hours serving them genuinely—not for the narcissistic satisfaction of helping, but because your dopamine system literally needs it.

Your cardiovascular system will thank you. Your brain chemistry will thank you. And the person you're helping will actually benefit while you experience euphoria through authentic service.

That's not altruism. That's evolution being remarkably kind.

Seva isn't sacrifice for others. It's self-preservation disguised as generosity.

CHAPTER 13: RIGHT ACTION (DHARMA)

The Moral Calculus Your Brain Is Constantly Running (Or: Why Cheating On That Exam Will Literally Age Your Brain)

You're in engineering college, facing the most competitive exam of your semester. Your friend whispers, "I've got the answer key. We could ace this." Your immediate reaction: pulse quickens, palms sweat, gut clenches. You *could* cheat. Objectively, the benefits are enormous—grades, scholarships, peer status, and less stress. The costs: zero enforcement risk (teachers don't check), nobody would know, minimal consequence if caught. By rational economic calculation, cheating is the optimal strategy.

Yet something inside says *no.* Not because you fear punishment. Not because of religious guilt. Something deeper. Your brain is experiencing two simultaneous computations: the cold rational calculation (cheating is optimal), and the moral intuition (cheating violates who you are). The conflict is agonizing.

Here's what neuroscience reveals: if you cheat despite this moral conflict, you literally create psychological damage—your brain interprets violating your own moral code as trauma, potentially causing what researchers call "moral injury"—the same neurological damage that affects soldiers who kill in violation of their values.

Dharma isn't about rules. It's about alignment—between your actions and your values, between individual benefit and collective wellbeing. Violating dharma creates biological stress that compounds over time.

Understanding this neurobiologically changes everything about how you approach "right action".

The Neuroscience of Moral Decision-Making (Or: Why Your Brain Has A Voting System)

Moral decisions activate distributed brain networks—not a single "morality region" but competing systems that must reconcile.

The Dual-Process Moral Brain: Emotion vs. Reason

When facing a moral dilemma, your brain activates two distinct systems that often conflict:

System 1 - The Emotional Route (Ventromedial Prefrontal Cortex, Amygdala):
This system responds quickly and intuitively. When you see someone suffering, or face betraying your values, this system activates immediately—before conscious reasoning.

The ventromedial prefrontal cortex (vmPFC) is involved in emotionally-driven moral decisions and generates rapid moral intuitions. The amygdala detects moral significance and emotional threat.

Example: Watching a friend be treated unfairly triggers immediate emotional response (anger, outrage) before you consciously deliberate.

System 2 - The Rational Route (Dorsolateral Prefrontal Cortex):
This system engages for utilitarian calculation—weighing costs, benefits, consequences.

The dorsolateral prefrontal cortex (dlPFC) handles reason-based moral judgments requiring conscious deliberation. This is where you calculate: "If I cheat, I gain ₹X utility, risk Y% punishment...".

Example: Deciding whether utilitarian logic justifies a rule violation requires slow, conscious reasoning.

The Reconciliation Problem:
These systems often conflict. Your emotional system says "this is wrong!" while your rational system says "but it maximizes my utility...".

Your brain must integrate these competing signals.

The anterior cingulate cortex (ACC) detects this conflict and attempts reconciliation. When conflict is severe, ACC activity increases dramatically—you experience the anguish of competing moral imperatives.

Intention, Harm, and Punishment: The Moral Decision Triplex

When judging whether an action is "right," your brain evaluates three dimensions:

1. Intention Assessment (Temporal Parietal Junction, Medial Prefrontal Cortex):
Did this person *intend* harm? The TPJ evaluates others' mental states, beliefs, intentions. An accidental harm is morally different from deliberate harm, even with identical outcomes.

Example: Hitting someone with a car accidentally vs. intentionally are morally distinct because intentions differ.

2. Harm Perception (Anterior Insula, Amygdala):
How much did this action harm others? The aINS detects suffering, and amygdala processes emotional significance. Greater harm = stronger moral disapproval.

Example: Stealing ₹100 is less morally egregious than stealing ₹1 lakh because harm differs.

3. Punishment Determination (Dorsolateral Prefrontal Cortex, Lateral Parietal Cortex):
What consequence is proportionate? The dlPFC integrates intention and harm to determine appropriate punishment.

These three systems interact: you understand intention (TPJ), perceive harm (aINS), integrate findings (dlPFC), and render moral judgment.

Moral Injury: When Violating Your Own Values Damages Your Neurobiology

Here's the critical discovery: when you act against your deeply-held moral values, your brain interprets this as violation—trauma.

Moral injury is defined as "psychological, social and spiritual suffering resulting from moral transgressions or violations of deeply-held moral beliefs and ethical standards". The core symptoms include:

- Shame and guilt: Not fear of punishment but self-directed condemnation
- Loss of trust: In yourself (if you could betray yourself, can you trust your own judgment?), in others (who encouraged betrayal?), in meaning systems that permitted betrayal
- Spiritual/existential crisis: Fundamental questioning of what's right

Secondary symptoms include depression, anxiety, anger, social alienation, relationship breakdown, self-harm.

The neurobiology: violating your own moral values triggers stress responses (cortisol, adrenaline) identical to threat responses. Your brain experiences this as danger because, fundamentally, moral violations are socially dangerous—communities punish moral transgressors.

Data from healthcare workers (a population experiencing high moral injury) show:

- 77% felt betrayed by institutions that violated their moral values
- 41.4% witnessed morally injurious events
- Those witnessing PMIEs showed 1.66× higher turnover intentions
- Those participating in PMIEs showed 1.38× higher burnout

The damage is measurable: moral injury is associated with depression, anxiety, PTSD, suicidal ideation, and decreased occupational functioning.

Crucially: this occurs regardless of external punishment. You can cheat without consequence, steal without arrest, betray without exposure—and still experience moral injury because *your own brain is punishing you for violating your values.*

Evolutionary Game Theory: Why Cooperation Seems Irrational But Is Actually Optimal

Here's where it gets elegant. Evolution selected for cooperation—for keeping moral commitments to yourself and others—because cooperation was *fitness-maximizing.*

The logic: imagine a population where everyone cheats when possible. What emerges? Complete defection—nobody cooperates, nobody trusts, nobody helps anyone. The society collapses.

Now imagine someone with the capacity to cooperate reliably. They seem worse off short-term (they cooperate while others defect). But over repeated interactions, over populations, cooperation-capable individuals accumulate allies, trust relationships, reciprocal help.

Result: cooperative individuals outsurvive defectors over long timescales. Humans evolved for cooperation—your moral intuitions exist because morality was survival advantage.

The kicker: evolution optimized your brain to experience moral transgression as painful precisely because that pain prevents cooperation-system breakdown. Your moral guilt serves biological function—it prevents you from doing things that would destroy your cooperative relationships.

Cheating on an exam *feels wrong* because evolution is begging you not to undermine the cooperative framework that kept your ancestors alive.

Real-World Applications: From Corporate Ethics to National Development

The Indian Dharma Crisis: Institutional Betrayal

India's moral injury epidemic is largely institutional rather than individual:

Healthcare workers: India's medical system creates daily moral injury:

- Pressured to see patients in 5 minutes (violates duty of care)
- Told to cut costs on necessary treatments (violates harm-prevention)
- Betrayed by institutions that recruited them with promises of ethical practice

Result: 63% of Indian medical professionals report burnout, with 22% experiencing symptoms consistent with moral injury.

Corporate professionals: Engineering/tech workers experience moral injury when:

- Pressured to cut corners on safety for profit
- Told to manipulate metrics/falsify data
- Ordered to implement products they believe are harmful
- Betrayed by organizations that preached ethics during hiring

Result: high attrition in ethical professionals (those with strong moral commitments), retention of those comfortable with moral compromise.

Government institutions: Bureaucrats and police experience moral injury when:

- Ordered to implement policies they believe are unjust
- Pressured to participate in corruption
- Betrayed by systems that promised impartial justice
- Forced to choose between personal integrity and employment

Result: massive burnout, corruption, cynicism, ineffectiveness.

The Economic Cost of Moral Injury

While difficult to quantify, the economic impact is enormous:

Healthcare: Turnover from moral injury costs approximately ₹5-10 lakh per physician (recruitment + training), multiplied by tens of thousands experiencing burnout.

Technology: Ethical engineers leaving companies represents intellectual capital loss. Companies known for moral compromise struggle to recruit top talent.

Government: Institutional moral injury creates cynicism, reduces public trust, enables corruption, undermines policy effectiveness.

The paradox: institutions causing moral injury for short-term profit create long-term destruction of their own functioning.

Emerging Solutions: Moral Repair

Recognizing moral injury has spawned interventions:

Organizational interventions:

- Psychological safety: Leaders must create environments where raising moral concerns is rewarded, not punished
- Just Culture: Investigating failures focusing on systems rather than individual blame—enabling honest moral discussion
- Transformative recognition: Publicly acknowledging wrongs and enabling moral repair

Individual interventions:

- Adaptive Disclosure: Processing moral transgressions through structured narrative
- Values-based behavioral activation: Recommitting to moral values through action
- Self-compassion practices: Counteracting shame/guilt patterns

Emerging data suggests these interventions measurably reduce moral injury symptoms and improve retention.

Critical Analysis: Debunking Dharma Myths

Myth 1: "Dharma Is Religious; It's Not Scientifically Relevant"

False. Dharma's core concept—alignment between values and action—is neurobiologically fundamental. Violating alignment creates measurable brain damage.

This isn't spiritual—it's neurobiological. Your brain experiences value misalignment as threat. The mechanism doesn't require belief in any deity.

Myth 2: "If Nobody Knows You Cheated/Lied/Betrayed, It Doesn't Matter"

Neurobiologically false. Moral injury originates from *your own recognition* of moral violation, not external consequences. Your brain knows. Your brain cares. Your brain suffers.

The person who cheats and gets away with it experiences internal moral injury—guilt, shame, loss of self-trust—even without detection.

Myth 3: "Utilitarianism—Maximum Good For Maximum People—Is Always Right"

Neurobiologically and ethically, false. Your emotional moral system evolved for a reason—it captures moral intuitions that pure utilitarian calculation misses.

Pure utilitarianism can justify atrocities. Your moral emotion system prevents this.

Right action requires both systems: emotional moral intuition *and* rational deliberation.

Myth 4: "I Can't Afford to Be Ethical; It'll Cost Me Success"

Research suggests otherwise. Ethical professionals who maintain moral boundaries often achieve greater long-term success than those who compromise.

Why? Because moral integrity enables trust. Reputation becomes invaluable. Communities reward moral agents.

Additionally, the psychological cost of moral injury—burnout, depression, lost trust—impairs future success.

How Western Morality Research Doesn't Apply to India

Much Western ethics research emphasizes individual moral autonomy—you get to choose your values and act accordingly.

India's reality: institutional hierarchies often *prevent* moral autonomy:

- You can't choose—you're ordered
- Refusing orders means employment termination
- Institutional pressure creates forced moral compromise

This explains India's extraordinary moral injury rates among professionals—forced value misalignment at scale.

Western solutions (individual ethical practices, personal resilience) address symptoms not causes. India's problem is institutional—requiring systemic change.

The Thought Experiment: Your Moral Boundary Map

Identify 5 potential situations where you might face value-action misalignment:

For each:

1. What value would be violated? (e.g., honesty, fairness, harm-prevention)
2. What pressure would push you to violate it? (career, money, social status)
3. How would you feel afterward? (guilt, shame, loss of self-trust)
4. What would be the long-term cost?

Most people discover that the short-term benefit of moral compromise is vastly outweighed by the long-term cost of moral injury.

A Simple Decision Protocol

When facing moral dilemma:

1. Identify the values in conflict: What are you being asked to compromise?

2. Consult both systems: What does your emotional moral intuition say? What does utilitarian calculation say?

3. Seek systems perspective: Is the pressure institutional? Is the institution corrupt or just misguided?

4. Evaluate long-term consequences: Would acting against your values cause moral injury? Would institutional participation enable further harm?

5. Choose alignment: Even if costly short-term, maintaining value-action alignment prevents long-term neurobiological damage.

This isn't idealistic. It's neurobiologically optimal.

Synthesis: Dharma As Development Strategy

For India's future, the dharma question is existential:

Do we build institutions that enable moral action or force moral compromise?

Current trajectory: institutional pressure forces value misalignment at scale. Result: epidemic moral injury, massive turnover, institutional dysfunction, brain drain.

Alternative trajectory: institutions that enable moral action, create psychological safety for ethical practice, reward dharma over compromise.

The neuroscience is clear: humans function optimally when aligned with their values. Forcing misalignment creates dysfunction, not efficiency.

Practical Actions for 2025

1. Personal dharma: Identify your core values. Make decisions honoring them.

2. Institutional accountability: When institutions pressure moral compromise, document, report, advocate for change.

3. Leadership dharma: If you lead, create psychological safety for moral discourse.

4. Professional integrity: Choose careers/organizations where your values align with mission.

5. Normalize moral discussion: Dharma isn't weakness; it's optimal functioning.

6. For India's future: Build institutions recognizing that moral alignment is prerequisite for health, productivity, and long-term success.

The Final Word (Or: Why Your Brain Knows Right Action Better Than Your Rationalizations)

Dharma isn't rule-following. It's alignment—between your deepest values and your actions, between individual wellbeing and collective flourishing.

Your brain evolved to experience moral integrity as deeply satisfying and moral violation as deeply damaging because evolution learned that cooperation-capable beings survived better than defectors.

When you feel moral conflict, you're not being weak. You're hearing 50,000 years of evolutionary wisdom telling you: "Your cooperation systems are at stake. Choose alignment."

The person who cheats and feels guilty isn't overreacting. They're experiencing an appropriate neurobiological alarm.

The person who maintains ethical integrity despite cost isn't naive. They're protecting their long-term psychological functioning and their evolutionary niche as a trustworthy cooperator.

For India's future, the question isn't whether to prioritize dharma. It's whether to listen to what your brain already knows: alignment is success.

Now close this chapter and ask: where are you compromising your values? What institutional pressure is creating misalignment? What would you need to realign?

Your brain is waiting for permission to stop experiencing moral conflict and start experiencing integrity.

Dharma isn't morality. It's optimal neurobiology in disguise.

CHAPTER 14: NON ATTACHMENT (VAIRAGYA)

The Happiness Treadmill That Neuroscience Explains (Or: Why Your BMW Will Make You Miserable In Exactly Three Months)

You spent three months earning enough to buy the car you've dreamed of since engineering college. The day you picked it up, you experienced pure euphoria—*finally*, you'd made it. For a solid week, your Instagram was flooded with photos of you in/with/near the BMW. Your WhatsApp status was a car selfie. You felt *successful.* Then week two: you noticed a scratch on the door. Week three: luxury car payments felt heavy every month. Week four: your friend bought a Tesla, and suddenly your BMW felt pedestrian. By month three, you were scrolling luxury SUVs wondering what you'd upgrade to next—the car that once represented pinnacle success now just felt... normal.

This isn't character weakness. It's neurobiology. It's called the hedonic treadmill, and it's why every achievement feels empty after a few months, why every possession loses its shine, and why billionaires are often miserable. Your brain is literally designed to return to baseline happiness regardless of external circumstances—a feature that helped ancestors survive trauma but makes modern consumption mindless.

Vairagya—non-attachment in Sanskrit—isn't about renouncing possessions or achieving ascetic poverty. It's about understanding your brain's hedonic adaptation so thoroughly that you *stop chasing temporary happiness through material acquisition.* It's about seeing the treadmill for what it is and stepping off.

Modern India is losing this wisdom precisely when Western science is rediscovering it. Let's talk about why your brain adapts to everything, and why the only sustainable happiness comes from what doesn't fade.

The Neuroscience of the Hedonic Treadmill (Or: Why Your Brain Is Fundamentally Optimistic And Essentially Pessimistic Simultaneously)

Evolution gave humans a peculiar gift: the ability to adapt to new circumstances. This was survival genius in ancestral environments. Predator attacks you? Survive the trauma through neurochemical desensitization. Famine ends? Stop celebrating—return to baseline vigilance.

The problem: the same mechanism that protects you from trauma also prevents you from benefiting from achievement.

The Hedonic Adaptation Mechanism: Three Pathways to Baseline

Research identifies three primary mechanisms through which your brain returns you to baseline happiness despite external circumstances:

1. Shifting Adaptation Levels:
When you get a salary raise, your initial happiness spike fades as you adjust to the new income level as your new "normal." You compare your current state to this new baseline rather than your previous state.

Neurologically, this involves your insula (interoceptive awareness) and anterior cingulate cortex (ACC) recalibrating reward thresholds. Dopamine—the reward neurotransmitter—doesn't increase permanently with higher income; instead, the *sensitivity* to dopamine changes. Your brain establishes new set points for comparison.

If you were earning ₹50 lakhs and felt wealthy, and now earn ₹100 lakhs, your brain doesn't maintain happiness levels. It recalibrates. ₹100 lakhs becomes the new neutral, and you feel happiness only when exceeding it (₹150 lakhs).

2. Desensitization:
Continuous exposure to stimulation reduces responsiveness. The luxury car you touch daily produces less dopamine than when new. The fancy

apartment you've lived in for 6 months feels normal.

This involves dopamine D2 receptor downregulation in your striatum—the pleasure center adapts to chronic stimulation by reducing receptor sensitivity. Technically, you're still experiencing the stimulus, but neurologically, you perceive it less.

3. Cognitive Reframing and Rationalization:
Your brain actively reinterprets circumstances to reduce their emotional impact. That promotion you were thrilled about? Your brain starts thinking, "Well, the responsibilities are actually quite stressful" or "I probably deserved it anyway".

This involves your prefrontal cortex actively reconstructing narratives, reducing the emotional salience of achievements. You're not consciously doing this—it's automatic meaning-making that neutralizes happiness.

The Happiness Set Point: Your Neurobiological Thermostat

Research across cultures and economic contexts shows that people maintain relatively stable happiness levels despite massive variation in wealth, possessions, or life circumstances.

Lottery winners experience initial euphoria, then return to pre-winning happiness levels within 6-12 months. People who become paralyzed adapt similarly—initial devastation fades, and happiness stabilizes at roughly their previous baseline.

This isn't universal—some people maintain higher set points, some lower—but the adaptation mechanism is consistent. Your brain has a happiness thermostat, and external changes prompt compensatory mechanisms returning you toward your set point.

The data: wealth and happiness correlation is approximately $r = 0.15$ across developed nations. Translation: income explains roughly 2% of happiness variation—98% comes from other factors.

The Material Treadmill: Why Materialism Specifically Kills Happiness

Here's the cruel discovery: materialism (prioritizing wealth and possessions) is uniquely demotivating compared to other value systems.

A large meta-analysis examining 753 effect sizes from 259 independent samples found that materialism shows negative correlation with well-being ($r = -0.19$ to -0.24). This means materialistic values *causally reduce* happiness, not just that unhappy people become materialistic.

Why materialism specifically?:

1. Extrinsic vs. Intrinsic Motivation: Materialism is extrinsic motivation (pursuing external validation through possessions). Happiness research shows that intrinsic goals (relationships, personal growth, contribution) produce lasting satisfaction, while extrinsic goals (wealth, status, appearance) produce hedonic adaptation.

2. Hedonic Adaptation Maximization: Possessions *maximally* trigger hedonic adaptation—you adapt to new purchases within months. Relationships, experiences, and personal growth adapt slowly or not at all.

3. Social Comparison Intensity: Materialism intensifies social comparison—you constantly compare your possessions to others' possessions. This comparison is inherently unsustainable; there's always someone wealthier, with better possessions.

4. Psychological Need Frustration: Materialism *undermines* satisfaction of basic psychological needs (autonomy, competence, relatedness) according to Self-Determination Theory. While pursuing possessions, you neglect relationships, autonomy, and mastery.

The result: materialistic individuals show lower life satisfaction, higher depression, worse relationships, and greater anxiety despite often earning more than non-materialistic peers.

Real-World Applications: From Corporate Burnout to Village Contentment

The Indian Paradox: Rising Income, Declining Happiness

India's economic growth over 25 years has created unprecedented wealth for millions. Yet happiness surveys show stagnant or declining life satisfaction among rising income groups.

A study of 80 males aged 40-50 earning 8-10 lakhs annually found that "happiness materialism" (belief that possessions create happiness) showed significantly negative correlation with life satisfaction ($r = -0.339$, $p < 0.01$). Success materialism didn't predict happiness, but happiness materialism *negatively predicted* life satisfaction.

Contributing factors in Indian context:

1. Status Anxiety: Rising incomes create new social classes with new comparisons. A ₹50 lakh earner in Bangalore compares themselves to ₹100 lakh earners (their newly visible peer group) and feels inadequate.

2. Hedonic Treadmill Acceleration: The pace of acquisition in urban India is frenzied—new car, house upgrade, luxury vacation planned. Each acquisition triggers treadmill adaptation then renewed seeking.

3. Work-Life Imbalance: Pursuing material accumulation requires work sacrifice—neglected relationships, missing family time, chronic stress.

4. Environmental Anxiety: Material consumption in India has environmental costs—water use for luxury goods, carbon emissions from consumption patterns. Subconsciously, materialists in polluted cities feel complicit.

The irony: the farmer in a village working ₹5 lakh annual income but embedded in relationships, community, traditions may show higher life satisfaction than the Bangalore executive earning ₹50 lakhs but atomized in corporate competition.

The Minimalism Movement: India's Counter-Culture

Simultaneously, India is witnessing counter-movements rejecting materialism:

Urban minimalism: Young professionals embracing tiny apartments, minimal possessions, experiential spending (travel, learning) over material accumulation.

Rural rediscovery: Some urbanites returning to villages, seeking simplicity after recognizing material pursuit's emptiness.

Spiritual resurgence: Yoga, meditation, vedic philosophy gaining traction among young Indians—explicitly non-materialist frameworks.

Research on minimalism shows measurable benefits:

- Stress reduction: Decluttering lowers cortisol levels by 75% in some studies
- Improved relationships: Less time managing possessions = more time with people
- Increased clarity: Reduced decision fatigue improves cognitive function
- Greater well-being: Minimalism shows positive correlation with well-being ($\beta = 0.13$, $p < 0.05$)

Young Indians adopting minimalism report feeling "liberated," "focused," and "less anxious" despite earning less than materialistic peers.

Tech Enabling Detachment: The Emerging Paradox

Ironically, Indian startups are building apps promoting non-attachment:

- Minimalist shopping lists: Apps limiting purchases, tracking spending, promoting intentional consumption
- Decluttering apps: Marie Kondo-style interfaces helping people release attachments
- Experience sharing: Apps prioritizing shared experiences over possession display
- Mindfulness-commerce: Platforms selling "simplicity" as product (which is ironic but effective in reaching digital natives)

The meta-irony: using consumerist technology to promote non-consumerism. Yet it's working—apps helping people reduce consumption receive millions of downloads.

Critical Analysis: Debunking Non-Attachment Myths

Myth 1: "Non-attachment Means Poverty or Deprivation"

Completely false. Non-attachment isn't about being poor or owning nothing. It's about releasing *emotional dependence* on possessions for identity/happiness.

You can own a nice home, a good car, quality clothes, and yet be non-attached—meaning these don't define you and their loss wouldn't devastate you.

Traditional Vairagya (Vedic non-attachment) wasn't renunciation. It was freedom—possessing things without being possessed *by* things.

Myth 2: "If You're Not Materialistic, You Won't Be Motivated"

False. Non-materialistic people show *higher* motivation for mastery, contribution, relationships. They work hard—just for different reasons.

An engineer pursuing mastery in programming is more motivated than one pursuing programmer status symbols. Non-materialists often show greater achievement than materialists because they're motivated by intrinsic factors sustaining attention over years.

Materialism actually *undermines* motivation—you adapt to acquisitions quickly, requiring constant new goals, creating exhaustion.

Myth 3: "Non-Attachment Is Giving Up"

Reframing needed: non-attachment is *optimization.* You're choosing to pursue happiness through paths with lower hedonic adaptation—relationships, growth, contribution.

Why chase possessions (hedonic adaptation = 3-6 months of happiness) when you could pursue relationships (minimal adaptation = decades of sustained happiness)?.

It's not giving up. It's getting smart.

Myth 4: "Western Research About Materialism Doesn't Apply To India"

Actually, it does. The hedonic treadmill is neurobiological—it operates identically in Mumbai as New York. Materialism's correlation with depression is consistent across cultures.

The Indian advantage: traditional wisdom about non-attachment is now being validated by Western neuroscience. India has 5,000 years of vairagya philosophy. The West just now discovered the brain mechanisms confirming it.

Rather than importing Western materialism, India could lead globally by *exporting non-attachment wisdom* backed by neuroscience.

The Thought Experiment: Your Possession-Happiness Audit

Track 5 possessions you own:

For each:

- How happy did you feel when acquiring it (1-10)?
- How happy are you feeling *now* with it (1-10)?
- How long did the happiness last?
- Would losing it devastate you?

Most people report:

- Initial happiness: 8-10
- Current happiness: 3-5
- Duration of peak happiness: 2-6 months
- Devastation risk: Moderate to low (most possessions aren't identity-defining)

This demonstrates hedonic adaptation empirically.

Now track 3 relationships:

- How happy do they make you feel (1-10)?
- Has happiness faded over time?
- How long have they sustained happiness?
- Would losing them devastate you?

Most report:

- Happiness: 7-9
- Fading: Minimal
- Duration: Years
- Devastation: High

This demonstrates why non-materialists pursue relationships—they produce sustained happiness.

A Simple 2-Week Experiment

Commit to 14 days of intentional non-attachment:

Week 1: Acquire nothing new. Notice the urge to purchase fade as hedonic adaptation releases.

Week 2: Declutter 10 items. Notice the psychological relief—cortisol drops, mental clarity improves.

Track your happiness, anxiety, focus, relationship quality daily.

Most people report measurable improvement—less anxiety, better sleep, stronger relationships, clearer thinking.

This demonstrates non-attachment's practical benefits within 2 weeks.

Synthesis: Non-Attachment As Development Strategy

For India's future, the hedonic treadmill has massive implications:

Economic Development: If materialism undermines happiness while consuming resources, can we redesign development around non-materialistic flourishing?.

Environmental Sustainability: Material consumption drives environmental degradation. Non-attachment reduces consumption while increasing well-being.

Mental Health: Depression, anxiety, burnout are epidemic in materialistically-driven economies. Non-attachment could be prevention.

Social Resilience: Communities with low materialism show stronger relationships, less inequality anxiety, better social cohesion.

The strategic opportunity: India could pioneer non-materialistic development—economic growth without consumption-driven environmental destruction.

Currently, India is importing Western materialism while abandoning Eastern non-attachment wisdom. The result: rising wealth, stagnant happiness, environmental crisis.

Practical Actions for 2025

1. Audit your materialism: Identify how much happiness you expect from possessions vs. actually receive.

2. Shift spending to experiences: Travel, learning, relationships produce lasting happiness; possessions produce temporary satisfaction.

3. Practice gratitude: Actively appreciate existing possessions rather than seeking new ones—this combats hedonic adaptation.

4. Embrace minimalism: Declutter intentionally. Notice the psychological relief. Maintain what brings joy; release what doesn't.

5. Invest in relationships: Time with loved ones is the highest-ROI happiness investment.

6. Redefine success: Not by possessions but by relationships, contribution, growth, experiences.

7. For India's future: Education should teach non-attachment alongside STEM. Career success without spiritual foundation creates empty high-achievers.

The Final Word (Or: Why Your Happiness Doesn't Actually Cost Money)

The most liberating discovery neuroscience has made about happiness is the simplest: your brain adapts to possessions quickly but adapts slowly to relationships, growth, and contribution.

This means the path to sustainable happiness doesn't require wealth. It requires wisdom.

The BMW will disappoint you. The relationship will sustain you. The promotion will adapt away. The mastery will compound. The vacation will fade. The learning will transform.

Your grandmother understood this. The Upanishads understood this. Neuroscience now confirms it.

Vairagya isn't mystical detachment. It's neurobiologically optimized life planning—pursuing what produces lasting happiness rather than what produces temporary pleasure.

For young Indians drowning in consumption-driven materialism, the ancient wisdom is suddenly modern: let go of the treadmill. Step onto solid ground. Pursue what genuinely sustains.

Your brain's hedonic thermostat will appreciate it.

So will your happiness.

Non-attachment isn't renouncing the world. It's refusing to be enslaved by it.

CHAPTER 10: FASTING

The Free Metabolic Reset Your Body Already Knows How To Do (Or: Why Not Eating Is Sometimes The Healthiest Thing You Can Eat)

Your grandmother fasts every *Ekadashi* (11th day of the lunar cycle), and your mother does *Karwa Chauth*. Your aunt follows *Navratri* fasting rituals. When you ask why, they say something vague about "spiritual purification" and "tradition." Meanwhile, your gym bro posts his intermittent fasting tracker on Instagram with hashtags like #16:8Protocol #MetabolicSwitching #BiohackingLife, claiming he's discovered revolutionary science that ancient Indians somehow never knew about. Your skeptical engineering brain sees both extremes and thinks: one side is religious dogma, the other is Silicon Valley narcissism.

Here's what neuroscience actually says: Both your grandmother and your gym bro are accidentally correct, just for different reasons. Fasting—periodic abstention from food—triggers something called metabolic switching: your body transitions from burning glucose (sugar) to burning fat and producing ketones, which activate cellular repair pathways, enhance brain function, improve insulin sensitivity, and extend lifespan in animal models.

Your grandmother didn't need peer-reviewed studies. Evolution figured this out millions of years ago when food scarcity was routine. Your body *expects* periods without food—it has entire genetic programs waiting to activate during fasting. Modern India's constant eating (breakfast, lunch, snacks, dinner, midnight maggi) never triggers these programs, leaving protective mechanisms dormant.

The irony: India invented fasting as spiritual practice 5,000 years ago. The West repackaged it as biohacking. Both work. Let's understand why.

The Neuroscience and Metabolism of Fasting (Or: What Happens When You Stop Feeding Your Cellular Energy Factory)

When you eat, your body runs on glucose. Between meals, it depletes glucose stores (glycogen in liver and muscles). After ~12-18 hours without food, something remarkable happens: metabolic switching—your body transitions from glucose metabolism to fat oxidation and ketone production.

The Metabolic Switch: From Glucose to Ketones

Under normal eating patterns (3 meals + snacks daily), you never run out of glucose. Your body remains in glucose-burning mode permanently. But during extended fasting (12-18+ hours), your liver glycogen depletes, forcing a metabolic pivot:

Stage 1 (0-12 hours): Glucose from recent meals and glycogen stores fuel your cells. Insulin levels remain elevated, signaling "fed state".

Stage 2 (12-18 hours): Glycogen depletes. Insulin drops. Glucagon (the hormone promoting fuel release) rises. Your body begins breaking down fat (lipolysis), releasing fatty acids.

Stage 3 (18+ hours): Ketogenesis activates. Your liver converts fatty acids into ketone bodies—primarily β-hydroxybutyrate (BHB). BHB becomes your brain's primary fuel, crossing the blood-brain barrier and powering neurons.

This isn't starvation. It's a programmed metabolic state your ancestors routinely entered. The difference: they didn't choose it; evolution selected for bodies that thrived during periodic food scarcity.

Autophagy: Your Body's Cellular Garbage Disposal

Here's where fasting gets genuinely magical (scientifically, not mystically). When insulin drops and mTOR (mechanistic target of rapamycin—a nutrient-sensing pathway) is inhibited, your cells activate autophagy—literally "self-eating".

Autophagy is cellular recycling. Your cells identify damaged proteins, dysfunctional mitochondria, and cellular debris, break them down, and recycle the components. It's like your body taking out the trash and composting it for new building materials.

Why this matters: autophagy declines with age and is impaired in neurodegenerative diseases (Alzheimer's, Parkinson's), cancer, and metabolic disorders. Fasting reactivates it.

Animal studies show fasting-induced autophagy clears toxic protein aggregates (like amyloid-beta in Alzheimer's), reduces inflammation, and extends lifespan. A 2024 review on intermittent fasting and neurodegeneration concluded: "IF influences a range of physiological mechanisms, including mitobiogenesis, autophagy, circadian rhythm alignment, and neuroinflammation".

Translation: periodic fasting literally cleans out your cellular junk.

BDNF and Neuroprotection: Why Fasting Makes Your Brain Sharper

β-hydroxybutyrate (BHB—the primary ketone) isn't just fuel. It's a signaling molecule activating neuroprotective pathways. Specifically, BHB increases brain-derived neurotrophic factor (BDNF)—a protein essential for neuron survival, growth, and synaptic plasticity.

BDNF is essentially miracle-gro for your brain. Higher BDNF = better memory, improved learning, enhanced neuroplasticity, protection against neurodegeneration. Fasting elevates BDNF significantly.

Additionally, ketones enhance mitochondrial function (your cellular powerhouses), reduce oxidative stress, and inhibit neuroinflammation. The result: fasting protects against age-related cognitive decline and neurodegenerative diseases.

A 2025 systematic review found intermittent fasting shows "substantial preventive and therapeutic potential" in Alzheimer's, Parkinson's,

Huntington's, and ALS.

Insulin Sensitivity: The Diabetes Connection

Here's the brutal metabolic reality: constant eating = constant insulin release = insulin resistance over time. Your cells become desensitized to insulin, requiring higher levels to achieve the same glucose uptake. This is the pathway to Type 2 diabetes.

Fasting reverses this. A meta-analysis of intermittent fasting in metabolic syndrome patients found:

- Fasting blood glucose reduced by 0.15 mmol/L ($p < 0.05$)
- HbA1c (long-term glucose marker) reduced by 0.08% ($p < 0.05$)
- Insulin levels reduced by 13.25 uUI ($p < 0.05$)
- HOMA-IR (insulin resistance marker) decreased by 0.31 ($p < 0.05$)
- Body weight reduced by 1.87 kg
- Waist circumference decreased by 2.08 cm

A 2025 randomized trial comparing 16:8 and 14:10 time-restricted eating to controls found:

- 16:8 group: 4.02% weight loss, fasting glucose declined 30.91 mg/dL, HbA1c reduced 0.499%
- 14:10 group: 3.15% weight loss, fasting glucose declined 28.06 mg/dL, HbA1c reduced 0.528%
- Control group: 0.55% weight loss, fasting glucose declined 9.09 mg/dL, HbA1c reduced 0.197%

Both fasting groups showed significantly greater improvements than controls.

The Circadian Connection: Why Timing Matters

Your body runs on circadian rhythms—24-hour biological cycles synchronized to light/dark patterns. Your metabolism follows these rhythms. Insulin sensitivity, glucose tolerance, and fat oxidation all peak at specific times.

Early time-restricted eating (eTRF)—eating within an early window (e.g., 8 AM to 5 PM)—aligns eating with your circadian metabolic peak.

Research shows eTRF produces superior benefits compared to late eating windows:

- Improved insulin sensitivity: A landmark study found eTRF improved β-cell responsiveness and insulin sensitivity despite participants fasting 18 hours before testing
- Better glucose tolerance: Morning glucose tolerance is superior to evening due to circadian rhythms
- Greater weight loss: Eating earlier in the day when metabolism is optimized enhances fat loss

A 2023 AHA presentation showed patients restricting eating to 10 hours daily (aligned with circadian rhythms) experienced:

- 3% weight reduction
- 4% waist circumference reduction
- 4% systolic blood pressure reduction
- 8% diastolic blood pressure reduction
- 11% LDL cholesterol reduction

The mechanism: eating aligns with circadian hormone release patterns, optimizing metabolism.

Real-World Applications: From Navratri to Silicon Valley

India's Fasting Traditions: Accidentally Optimized Protocols

Indian fasting practices—Ekadashi, Karwa Chauth, Navratri, Ramadan—unintentionally implemented intermittent fasting protocols validated by modern research:

Ekadashi (biweekly 24-hour fasts): Roughly 16:8 or 20:4 intermittent fasting. Triggers metabolic switching, activates autophagy, improves insulin sensitivity.

Navratri (9-day modified fasting): Participants eat specific foods (fruits, nuts, limited grains) at restricted times. This is essentially time-restricted eating with nutrient composition changes.

Ramadan (dawn-to-dusk fasting): Classic intermittent fasting. A month-long protocol providing sustained metabolic benefits.

The brilliance: these traditions created adherence through

cultural/religious meaning. You don't need willpower when fasting is spiritually significant. Modern "biohackers" struggle with compliance; traditional Indians fasted for millennia because culture embedded it.

The Indian Diabetes Epidemic: Fasting as Intervention

India has 77 million diabetics—the second-highest globally. Type 2 diabetes is epidemic among urban populations. Fasting offers accessible intervention:

Studies specifically examining intermittent fasting in Indian Type 2 diabetics show:

- Significant reductions in fasting glucose and HbA1c
- Improved insulin sensitivity and reduced insulin resistance
- Weight loss and visceral fat reduction
- Better adherence compared to continuous caloric restriction

A 2025 review concluded: "Intermittent fasting is recommended as a viable first-line strategy for managing T2DM, especially for individuals with obesity and insulin resistance".

For a nation struggling with diabetes and limited healthcare access, fasting is free, culturally embedded, and evidence-based.

Corporate Wellness and Productivity

Indian startups are beginning to recognize fasting's productivity benefits. Ketones enhance cognitive function—clearer thinking, better focus, sustained energy without glucose crashes.

Anecdotally, engineers report peak coding performance during fasted states. The mechanism: stable ketone fuel + enhanced BDNF + reduced inflammatory cytokines = optimized brain function.

Some companies are implementing "fasting-friendly" workplace cultures—no pressure to attend breakfast meetings, respecting employees' eating windows.

Critical Analysis: Debunking Fasting Myths

Myth 1: "Fasting Slows Your Metabolism"

False. Short-term fasting (up to 48-72 hours) *increases* metabolic rate through norepinephrine release. Your body doesn't enter "starvation mode" after missing breakfast.

Long-term chronic caloric restriction can slow metabolism. Intermittent fasting doesn't—you're eating the same calories, just in a compressed window.

Myth 2: "You'll Lose Muscle Mass"

Partially false. Fasting preserves muscle better than continuous caloric restriction when protein intake is adequate. Growth hormone increases during fasting, protecting lean mass.

However, *extended fasting without resistance training* can cause muscle loss. The solution: maintain protein intake during eating windows and continue strength training.

Myth 3: "Breakfast Is The Most Important Meal"

This was marketing, not science. The "breakfast is essential" narrative originated from cereal companies. Research shows skipping breakfast (when done as part of time-restricted eating) doesn't harm health and may improve metabolic markers.

What matters: *when* you eat relative to your circadian rhythm, not whether you eat breakfast specifically.

Myth 4: "Fasting Is Dangerous For Everyone"

False. Fasting is safe for most healthy adults. However, it's contraindicated for:

- Pregnant/breastfeeding women
- Children and adolescents (still growing)
- People with eating disorders
- Individuals with certain medical conditions (consult physician)

For Type 2 diabetics on medication, fasting requires medical supervision to avoid hypoglycemia.

Myth 5: "All Fasting Protocols Are Equivalent"

False. Timing matters enormously. Early time-restricted eating (eTRF) aligned with circadian rhythms produces superior benefits compared to late eating.

Eating 12 PM - 8 PM (late window) shows fewer benefits than 8 AM - 4 PM (early window) for glucose control and insulin sensitivity.

How Western Research Doesn't Apply to Indian Conditions

Most fasting research uses Western populations with different baseline diets, activity levels, and genetic factors:

Dietary composition: Indians consume higher carbohydrate loads (rice, roti) than Western diets. Fasting's glucose benefits may be more pronounced in high-carb populations.

Genetic factors: South Asians show higher diabetes susceptibility at lower BMI. Fasting interventions may need adaptation for this genetic context.

Cultural compliance: Indians have millennia of fasting tradition. Adherence may be higher than Western populations unfamiliar with fasting.

The Thought Experiment: Your Personal Metabolic Switch

Track your eating window for one week:

Current pattern: Note first bite to last bite daily. Most people eat over 14-16 hours.

Metabolic analysis: If you eat over 12+ hours daily, you're never triggering metabolic switching. Your body remains in glucose-burning mode constantly.

Intervention design: Choose a protocol:

- 16:8: Fast 16 hours, eat 8 hours (e.g., 12 PM - 8 PM or better: 8 AM - 4 PM)
- 14:10: Fast 14 hours, eat 10 hours (easier compliance)
- Alternate-day fasting: Eat normally one day, fast (or 500-600 calories) the next

Measurement: Track energy, focus, sleep, weight, mood for 4 weeks.

Most people report improved energy, mental clarity, and modest weight loss within 2-4 weeks.

Synthesis: Fasting As India's Most Underutilized Health Tool

For a nation facing epidemic diabetes, obesity, neurodegenerative disease, and healthcare infrastructure limitations, fasting is remarkably well-suited:

It's free: No cost, no prescription needed.

It's culturally embedded: India has fasting traditions spanning millennia.

It's evidence-based: Robust research demonstrates metabolic, neurological, and longevity benefits.

It's scalable: Unlike pharmaceutical interventions requiring distribution infrastructure, fasting requires only education.

The challenge: modernization is eroding traditional fasting practices while importing Western constant-eating patterns. Urban Indians now eat constantly—snacks, meals, late-night food—never triggering the metabolic programs evolution designed.

Practical Actions for 2025

1. Start small: Begin with 12:12 (12-hour fast, 12-hour eating window). Gradually extend to 14:10 or 16:8.

2. Align with circadian rhythms: Eat earlier in the day when metabolism is optimized. Avoid late-night eating.

3. Maintain nutrition quality: Fasting isn't permission to eat junk during eating windows. Focus on whole foods, adequate protein.

4. Monitor health markers: Track fasting glucose, HbA1c, weight, energy levels.

5. Respect contraindications: Consult physicians if diabetic, pregnant, or managing chronic conditions.

6. Leverage cultural traditions: Use Ekadashi, Navratri, or personal spiritual frameworks for adherence.

7. For India's future: Normalize fasting as evidence-based health practice, not just religious observance. Integrate into medical recommendations for diabetes and metabolic syndrome.

The Final Word (Or: Why Your Grandmother's Ekadashi Was Biohacking Before Silicon Valley Existed)

Fasting isn't new. It's ancient. Your body evolved expecting periodic food scarcity and developed entire metabolic programs to thrive during these periods.

Modern constant eating—breakfast, snacks, lunch, chai, dinner, midnight maggi—is the evolutionary novelty. Your body doesn't know what to do with 16-hour eating windows. It's waiting for the fast that never comes, unable to activate autophagy, metabolic switching, or neuroprotection.

The neuroscience is unequivocal: periodic fasting enhances insulin sensitivity, activates cellular repair, protects brain function, and extends healthspan.

Your grandmother knew this intuitively. The Vedic sages knew this philosophically. Evolution knew this biologically.

Now you know it scientifically.

The beautiful irony: India invented fasting as spiritual practice, then forgot its metabolic benefits while importing Western constant-eating patterns. Meanwhile, Silicon Valley "discovered" intermittent fasting and sells it back to Indians as innovation.

The circle completes when science validates tradition.

Now close this chapter, stop eating after 6 PM tonight, and don't eat again until 10 AM tomorrow. Track how you feel. Notice the mental clarity around hour 14. Recognize the sustained energy without glucose crashes.

That's not deprivation. That's your evolutionary heritage finally activating.

Fasting isn't starvation. It's your body remembering how it was designed to function.

Congratulations! If you made it to the end of this book without tossing it out the window, doom-scrolling Instagram, or joining a raw-food startup, you officially have more focus and curiosity than the average caffeinated engineering student at 2 AM.

If you found yourself snorting at the jokes, nodding at the science, or feeling just a little bit smarter (or at least a lot more Indian), don't stop here. Science-y irreverence and Indian cultural mashups are my jam—and, yes, I write more books in this style.

To fuel your next reading binge, check out other books by Rajat Akre—available on Amazon (because let's be honest, nobody is waiting for Flipkart delivery right now):

Browse Rajat Akre's books on Amazon (https://www.amazon.in/s?i=stripbooks&rh=p_27%3ARajat%2BAkre&ref=dp_byline_sr_book_1)

Go ahead—click, browse, and gift at least one to your friend who forwards WhatsApp 'miracle cure' messages (you both know who I mean).

May your dopamine spikes always be evidence-based, and your bookshelf never run out of good science.

Now, what are you waiting for? Science waits for no one (but Amazon will ship within three days).

ABOUT THE AUTHOR

Rajat Akre is a designer, teacher, and unapologetic philosopher from Nagpur, India.
Armed with a Master's in Design from IIITDM Jabalpur and an engineering degree he politely ignores, he's spent the last few years teaching design thinking, UX, and creative chaos at institutes like MIT Institute of Design, Avantika University, and Symbiosis School of Design.

He founded Inizio Design Studio, where ideas, not budgets, decide creativity. When he's not teaching students how to prototype or philosophize, he's decoding the Upanishads in meme language, trading stocks like they're karmic lessons, or finding beauty in contradictions, sunlight and sarcasm, silence and deadlines.

Rajat believes wisdom should be open-source and enlightenment should never come with GST. This book (like most of his work) is a protest against the myth that you have to buy peace. You only pay for printing; the truth remains free.

You may reach out to him on rajatakre@gmail.com

www.ingramcontent.com/pod-product-compliance
Ingram Content Group UK Ltd.
Pitfield, Milton Keynes, MK11 3LW, UK
UKHW011513190726
13845UKWH00034B/1245

9 789334 456103